T0269172

The Innate Immune System

Dedication

**For Marianne, without you none of this would happen.
For Matthew, Rhiannon, Cleo, and Elsa, you will never be
in anyone's shadow – follow your dreams.**

The Innate Immune System

A compositional and functional perspective

Tom P. Monie
Christ's College and Institute of Continuing Education
University of Cambridge, United Kingdom

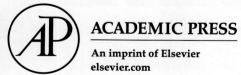

ELSEVIER

ACADEMIC PRESS

An imprint of Elsevier
elsevier.com

Academic Press is an imprint of Elsevier
125 London Wall, London EC2Y 5AS, United Kingdom
525 B Street, Suite 1800, San Diego, CA 92101-4495, United States
50 Hampshire Street, 5th Floor, Cambridge, MA 02139, United States
The Boulevard, Langford Lane, Kidlington, Oxford OX5 1GB, United Kingdom

Notices
Knowledge and best practice in this field are constantly changing. As new research and experience
broaden our understanding, changes in research methods, professional practices, or medical
treatment may become necessary.

Practitioners and researchers may always rely on their own experience and knowledge in
evaluating and using any information, methods, compounds, or experiments described herein.
In using such information or methods they should be mindful of their own safety and the safety
of others, including parties for whom they have a professional responsibility.

To the fullest extent of the law, neither the Publisher nor the authors, contributors, or editors,
assume any liability for any injury and/or damage to persons or property as a matter of products
liability, negligence or otherwise, or from any use or operation of any methods, products,
instructions, or ideas contained in the material herein.

Library of Congress Cataloging-in-Publication Data
A catalog record for this book is available from the Library of Congress

British Library Cataloguing-in-Publication Data
A catalogue record for this book is available from the British Library

ISBN: 978-0-12-804464-3

For information on all Academic Press publications visit our website at
https://www.elsevier.com/books-and-journals

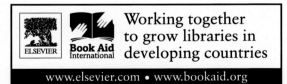

Working together
to grow libraries in
developing countries

www.elsevier.com • www.bookaid.org

Publisher: Sara Tenney
Acquisition Editor: Linda Versteeg-Buschmann
Editorial Project Manager: Halima Williams
Production Project Manager: Edward Taylor
Designer: Mark Rogers

Typeset by TNQ Books and Journals

Contents

Preface ix
Acknowledgments xiii

1. A Snapshot of the Innate Immune System

1.1 **A Brief History of Immunity** 1
    1.1.1 The Rise of Innate Immunity 4
    1.1.2 Self, Nonself, and the "Danger" Hypothesis 7
1.2 **The Immune System—A Complex Defense System** 10
1.3 **Functional Elements on the Innate Immune Response** 13
    1.3.1 Barrier Functions 15
    1.3.2 Immune Tissues 16
    1.3.3 Immune Cells 17
    1.3.4 Protein and Peptide Defenses 22
    1.3.5 Cell Death 25
1.4 **The Mucosa-Associated Innate Immune System** 26
    1.4.1 The Cells of the Gastrointestinal Tract Epithelium and Their Role in Innate Defense Mechanisms 27
    1.4.2 Peyer's Patches and M Cells 28
    1.4.3 Secreted Defenses 28
1.5 **Additional Homeostatic Functions Involved in Innate Immune Responses** 36
    1.5.1 The Heat Shock Response 36
    1.5.2 The Unfolded Protein Response 36
    1.5.3 Autophagy 36
    References and Further Reading 38

2. Immune Cells and the Process of Pattern Recognition

2.1 **The Cellular Basis of the Innate Immune System** 41
    2.1.1 Monocytes 42
    2.1.2 Macrophages 42
    2.1.3 Dendritic Cells 46
    2.1.4 Neutrophils 47
    2.1.5 Eosinophils 52
    2.1.6 Mast Cells and Basophils 54
    2.1.7 Innate Lymphoid Cells 55
    2.1.8 Gamma-Delta (γδ) T Cells 58

2.2   **Pattern Recognition Receptor Signaling Pathways**   59
        2.2.1   Pattern Recognition Receptors Recognize Exogenous
                and Endogenous Dangers   59
        2.2.2   Domain Organization of the Pattern Recognition
                Receptors   61
        2.2.3   Toll-Like Receptor Signaling   62
        2.2.4   C-Type Lectin Receptor Signaling   70
        2.2.5   Cytoplasmic Pattern Recognition Receptors   73
        2.2.6   Nucleotide-Binding, Leucine-Rich Repeat-Containing
                Receptor Signaling   73
        2.2.7   Nucleic Acid–Sensing Immune Receptors in the
                Cytoplasm   77
        References and Further Reading   79

3. **Effector Mechanisms and Cellular Outputs**

    3.1   **Cytokines**   83
            3.1.1   The Interleukin-1 Family   84
            3.1.2   The Tumor Necrosis Factor Families   87
            3.1.3   The Interferon Family   87
            3.1.4   Interleukin-6 and Interleukin-8   89
            3.1.5   The Key Antiinflammatory Cytokines:
                    Interleukin-4, -5, -10, and -13   92
            3.1.6   The Interleukin-17 Family, Interleukin-21, and
                    Interleukin-22   92
            3.1.7   Additional Immune-Related Cytokines   93
    3.2   **Acute Phase Proteins and the Acute Phase Response**   94
    3.3   **Reactive Oxygen Species**   97
    3.4   **Enzymatic Cascades and Enzymatic Activation**   98
            3.4.1   Blood Coagulation Pathways   98
            3.4.2   Eicosanoids   99
            3.4.3   Complement   100
            3.4.4   Caspases   107
    3.5   **Cell Death**   109
            3.5.1   Apoptosis   110
            3.5.2   Necrosis   113
            3.5.3   Necroptosis   114
            3.5.4   Pyroptosis   116
            References and Further Reading   116

4. **Integrated Innate Immunity—Combining Activation
    and Effector Functions**

    4.1   **The Detection of Bacterial Lipopolysaccharide**   121
            4.1.1   Activation of TLR4 Signaling by Extracellular
                    Lipopolysaccharide   123
            4.1.2   The TLR4 Signaling Pathway   126
            4.1.3   Intracellular Lipopolysaccharide Is Detected by
                    Members of the Inflammatory Caspases   130

4.2   Interleukin 1β Is Produced Following Activation of the
        Inflammasome   130
        4.2.1   Activation of the Inflammasome   132
        4.2.2   Protein Interactions Drive Assembly of the Inflammasome   140
        4.2.3   Regulation of the Inflammasome Is Important   141
4.3   The Innate Response to Bacterial Infection With *Salmonella*   144
        4.3.1   Salmonellosis   144
        4.3.2   *Salmonella* Is Recognized by a Range of Innate Immune
                Components   145
        4.3.3   *Salmonella*-Derived Lipoproteins Stimulate TLR2-Driven
                Inflammatory Signaling   146
        4.3.4   Flagellin Is a Major Immune Stimulus   149
        4.3.5   Extracellular Flagellin Is Detected by TLR5   149
        4.3.6   Intracellular Flagellin and Components of the
                Type III Secretion System Activate the NAIP/NLRC4
                Inflammasome   153
4.4   Innate Recognition and the Response to the *Influenza* Virus   155
        4.4.1   The Influenza A Virus Replication Cycle   156
        4.4.2   Antigenic Drift and Antigenic Shift in Influenza A Virus   159
        4.4.3   Influenza A Virus and the Innate Immune Response   159
        4.4.4   Evasion of the Innate Immune Response by Influenza
                A Virus   164
      References and Further Reading   164

5.   **Connecting the Innate and Adaptive Immune Responses**

5.1   **The Transcriptional Regulation of MHC Class I and II Genes**   171
        5.1.1   NLRC5 and the Transcription of MHC Class I Genes   172
        5.1.2   CIITA and the Transcription of MHC Class II Genes   174
5.2   **Complement and the Adaptive Immune Response**   175
        5.2.1   Complement and the Function of B Cells   175
        5.2.2   Complement and the T-Cell Response   177
5.3   **Autophagy and the Development of T and B Cells**   178
5.4   **The Dendritic Cell Is the Interface Between the Innate
        and the Adaptive Immune Response**   179
        5.4.1   Dendritic Cells and Their Interaction With T Cells   181
5.5   **Adjuvants, PRRs, and Vaccination**   183
        5.5.1   Licensed Adjuvants and the Hunt for New Ones   183
        5.5.2   Adjuvants and PRRs   184
      References and Further Reading   185

6.   **The Innate Immune System in Health and Disease**

6.1   **Inflammation and Atherosclerosis**   189
6.2   **Rheumatoid Arthritis**   192
        6.2.1   The Initiation and Establishment of Rheumatoid Arthritis   194
        6.2.2   The Role of Cytokines in the Pathogenesis of Rheumatoid
                Arthritis   195
        6.2.3   Rheumatoid Arthritis, Pattern Recognition Receptors,
                and Therapy   195

6.3   Autoinflammatory Syndromes   196
    6.3.1   Familial Mediterranean Fever   197
    6.3.2   Cryopyrin-Associated Periodic Syndromes   198
    6.3.3   Macrophage Activation Syndrome   199
    6.3.4   Autoinflammatory Syndromes Can Result From
           Defects in IL-1 Family Member Antagonists   199
    6.3.5   Treatment of Periodic Inflammatory Disorders   201
6.4   Inflammatory Bowel Disease   202
6.5   Animal Models of Inflammatory Disorders   203
    References and Further Reading   206

Index   209

Preface

Without an innate immune system you would not be in a position to read this book, and I would not have been able to write it. Our bodies face a near continual bombardment of molecules and pathogens with the potential to cause extensive cellular damage and destruction. It is the job of the innate immune response to provide immediate and unwavering protection. It is a beautiful and complex example of biological engineering that allows us to not only survive but also actually prosper in biologically hostile environments.

Could one describe the innate immune response as the most important of our many biological systems? Maybe not, as there are physiological processes whose absence would be more rapidly fatal. However, the innate immune system is certainly one of the most important and, at least in my slightly biased view, one of the most interesting. In part, this is due to the fact that we are still rapidly learning more and more about what the innate immune system actually is and how it functions in both health and disease. It also stems from the fascinating approaches used by the innate immune system to ensure that it responds in a balanced, appropriate, and regulated manner.

Aimed at students studying the field of immunology from a biological or a medical perspective, or researchers needing an overview or refresher on innate immune function, this textbook will introduce you to the main functional elements of the innate immune response, before highlighting how they work to protect against bacterial and viral infection. The connection between the innate and the adaptive arms of the immune defenses will be briefly touched on and highlight how the innate immune response can actually be an important, or even the major, contributor to the development of long-term chronic illness. It never was, and never will, provide a fully comprehensive and encyclopedic coverage of the innate immune response. It will, however, enthuse and inform, interest and educate, and allow you, as the reader, to identify areas of innate immunity that you want to follow up in a more comprehensive and detailed manner. To this end, each section is accompanied by a brief selection of related references and further reading to allow you to choose and develop your own interests.

I began my own undergraduate education in the early days of the innate immune revolution that followed from Charles Janeway's theories on pattern recognition. Until that point, teaching and research in immunology had been almost completely focused on elements of the adaptive immune response such as antibodies, the role of the major histocompatibility complex, T cells, and B cells. Although innate components, such as the complement system, were well understood, the area of innate immunology bore no relation to the field as we know it today. Maybe this was why I remember saying to a colleague, "I can't stand immunology. There's no way I'll ever be an immunologist." I am clearly not a fortune teller, and while I will never view myself as a classical immunologist, more of a protein biochemist really, it is without doubt the intricacies of the innate immune system and in particular the processes around pattern recognition that now drive and motivate me. That this book exists is testament to the fact that one's younger self does not always know best and that science has a tendency to always throw out some surprises.

Despite the explosion of research into the innate immune system, I have never really felt that this has been reflected in the range and repertoire of immunology textbooks available to students studying modern day immunology. There are a number of excellent immunology textbooks that give strong prominence to the innate immune system. Many more textbooks, however, focus on the adaptive response and only make brief mention of the innate elements. A desire to, at least in part, redress some of this imbalance was one of the primary motivations to write this book as was the wish to make available to students the sort of textbook that I myself would have liked to have available over the years as I explored and learned more about the innate immune response.

I have often found that I come across a new area of interest, a new immune system, or a new signaling cascade, only to discover that there are gaps in my previous knowledge that need filling before I can really appreciate and understand the new areas. It is this experience that lies behind the structuring of the book. As a reader I envisage two primary ways in which the book will be used. In one case you, as the reader, will dip in and out of the parts that interest you or are most relevant to your current work and study. Alternatively, for those like myself who find themselves beginning their innate immune journey somewhat overwhelmed by its vastness, I suggest starting at the beginning. This will allow you to be briefly and gradually introduced to the main players, processes, and components, which together comprise the major elements of the innate immune response. Armed with an understanding of these elements, you will be primed to move on and explore the more detailed examples in this work and the wider immune field.

As with all pieces of work in a rapidly moving research field, particularly one with both time and size constraints, I was never going to be able to cover all areas of innate immunity with the level of breadth and depth I might have wanted. Rather unsurprisingly, therefore, this first edition sees something of a bias toward the areas of innate immunity that have interested me most over the course of my research career so far. I hope with time to be able to expand on those areas that have received little more than superficial coverage, update those that continue to rapidly progress, and broaden the scope and depth of the specific examples. No doubt, there will also be completely new areas to incorporate to continue to highlight the diversity and the beauty of the innate immune response.

On a final note, enjoy the book, find it useful and who knows, maybe you too will one day be turned into an immunologist!

Tom P. Monie

Acknowledgments

Writing acknowledgments and giving speeches are both similar in that one gets them finished and only then realizes that something or someone critical has been left out. I will be upfront in my apologies to anyone who feels they have been missed out. This is not due to any lack of appreciation on my part, but simply due to my own incompetence in remembering everyone who has helped in some form along the way. To minimize this likelihood I have decided for now to keep these acknowledgments succinct and targeted to those that had a dramatically direct influence or impact, whether they know it or not. Here goes. Jane Greatorex and Andrew Lever, without whom I would never have started down this whole route many years ago; Nick Gay, who first got me interested in innate immunity and whose unwavering support has helped shape my career; Clare Bryant, with whom many hours of innate immune chat have passed and who has helped nurture my love of the nucleotide-binding, leucine-rich repeat–containing receptors; to the teams of researchers in biochemistry and the vet school with whom many thoughts and ideas have been discussed over the years, but particularly my own students Joe Boyle, Sophie Mayle, and Rhiannon Parkhouse; Jonathan Powell for taking a punt and letting me follow my interests; my production and editorial team, especially Linda Versteeg-Buschman for getting me involved and Halima Williams for the gentle prodding to keep me (mainly) on track; Thomas Kufer, for the understanding and offers of help in the hard times; and Marianne, for putting up with the long evenings, late nights, and early mornings while this was all written. Thank you all.

Section 1

A Snapshot of the Innate Immune System

1.1 A BRIEF HISTORY OF IMMUNITY

It is hard to pinpoint a precise time in history that saw the birth of immunology as a field of scientific research. A range of individuals have contributed to the key experiments that have led initially to our awareness and subsequently our ever-improving understanding of immune function. This has included, for example, work on vaccination, phagocytosis, complement, antibodies, T and B cell function, and pattern recognition (Fig. 1.1). On occasion these pieces of work and experimentation have led to radical or even paradigm shifts in the accepted viewpoint, theories, and mechanisms of immunology. The significance of some of this work only sometimes becomes apparent either much later or following further study.

In many ways the pioneering work of Edward Jenner at the end of the 18th century presents the most obvious point at which begins the story of immunology. Jenner had made the observation that milkmaids very rarely appear to become infected with smallpox, which was a major cause of both mortality and morbidity. He suspected that this was because they often caught the highly similar, but much less pathogenic, disease cowpox from the animals they were tending. To test his theory, Jenner used material extracted from a cowpox lesion from a milkmaid's hand to inoculate a young boy called James Phipps. Six weeks later, Jenner then infected Phipps with smallpox using material obtained from a lesion. Fortunately for Phipps, Jenner's theory proved accurate and the young boy failed to develop smallpox—he had been successfully vaccinated and provided with lifelong protection against the disease. Although there was much resistance and fear of Jenner's approach, the process of using cowpox inoculation to protect against smallpox gradually became more widespread and just less than 200 years later in 1978, following a global vaccination program, smallpox was successfully eradicated. Although Jenner knew very little about how his cowpox inoculum protected against infection, it represented the beginning of vaccination against a wide range of pathogens and as research in this field developed, it became increasingly obvious that the immune system was the key player driving this protection. Successful vaccination requires activation of two different types of immune response—the innate response and the adaptive response (Fig. 1.2) (Section 5).

The Innate Immune System. http://dx.doi.org/10.1016/B978-0-12-804464-3.00001-6

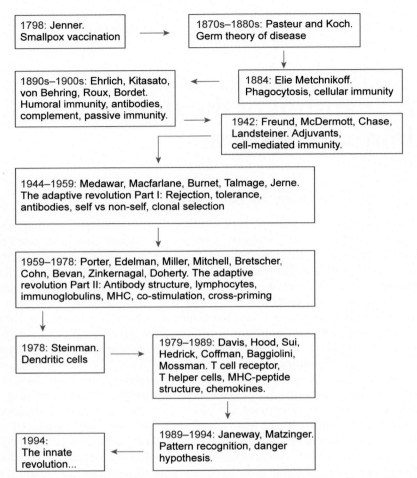

FIGURE 1.1 **An immunological timeline.** A brief summary of selected key milestones, discoveries, individuals, and pieces of work that were critical to the development and progression of immunological research and thinking. The list is far from exhaustive.

Toward the latter part of the 19th century, rapid progress was made in identifying and explaining a number of the key paradigms that proceeded to drive immunological research through the 20th century and still continue to do so today (Fig. 1.1). This included the work of Koch and Pasteur, two intense scientific rivals, whose combined efforts in the field of microbiology led to the development of the germ theory of disease and therefore provided a rational explanation for the success of Jenner's smallpox vaccinations. This was complemented through the demonstration by Von Behring and Kitasato that serum could be used to transfer protection from one host to another. They showed that soluble elements of the serum could protect against disease and

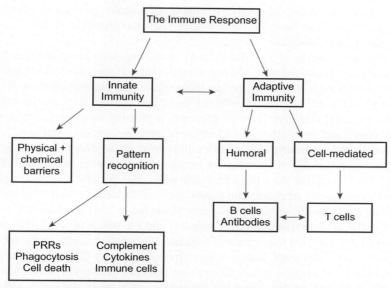

FIGURE 1.2   The Immune System. A schematic representation of the separation of the immune system into its innate and adaptive components in which key processes are isolated and identified.

hence laid the foundation for passive immunization. Their work on diphtheria led to Von Berhing being awarded the Nobel Prize for Physiology and Medicine in 1901. It also stimulated the work of Paul Ehrlich who proposed that the protective soluble elements were specific molecules or immune bodies, which we now recognize as antibodies, and that these were secreted from certain cells following their specific stimulation. Also around this time, Elie Metchnikoff introduced the scientific world to the concept of phagocytosis. Working with starfish larvae, he observed that certain cell types were able to ingest and internalize particles of dye or fragments of splinters that had been introduced into the larvae. He coined the term "phagocytes" to describe these cells and was able to demonstrate their importance in providing the early stages of protection against bacterial disease. Ehrlich and Metchnikoff were jointly awarded the Nobel Prize for Physiology and Medicine in 1908 "in recognition of their work on immunity." Immunology had well and truly taken off.

Despite the fact that Metchnikoff had clearly demonstrated the importance of phagocytic cells in fighting infection, it was the humoral—the cell-free, soluble component—of the immune response that dominated immunological thinking until the outbreak of the Second World War. This was led by further work to understand how antibodies conferred protective immunity and also by research that highlighted the contribution of antibody to the immunopathology of conditions, such as anaphylactic shock and hemolytic anemia. Complement also joined the family of soluble mediators of immune protection following the groundbreaking work by Jules Bordet, winner of the 1919 Nobel Prize in Physiology and Medicine.

The contribution of specific cells in conferring immune protection had, however, not been forgotten, and experiments that transferred cells from guinea pigs immunized with *Mycobacterium tuberculosis* to naive animals showed that the cells were, in fact, able to induce a protective immune response on subsequent bacterial challenge. Hence, there was a growing awareness of both the importance and the mechanisms of action of antibody-mediated (humoral) and cell-mediated immunity. This led to a rapid period of discovery in which many of the key principles of the adaptive immune response were established (Fig. 1.1). These included the structure of antibodies, the identification of lymphocytes as mediators of cellular immunity, the elucidation of clonal selection to explain antibody diversity, the discovery of the major histocompatibility complex (MHC), understanding of the genetics and the ontogeny of the adaptive immune defenses, the importance of tolerance, and greater clarity on the recognition of self and nonself. Many of these areas of immunity fall well and truly in the remit of the adaptive arm of the immune response. Some will be touched on briefly in Section 5 when I consider the interaction between the innate and the adaptive responses, and all are comprehensively covered in the resources listed in References and Further Reading at the end of this section.

1.1.1 The Rise of Innate Immunity

The adaptive immune response and the role of B and T lymphocytes, antibodies, MHC, and the like, completely dominated immunology until the end of the 1980s. At this point, Charles Janeway gave a seminal address at the Cold Spring Harbor Symposium on Immune Recognition entitled "Approaching the asymptote? Evolution and revolution in immunology." In this address, Janeway highlighted the fact that T and B cells do not produce good immune responses against purified proteins, but require the presence of an adjuvant such as complete Freund's adjuvant, which is a suspension of heat-killed *Mycobacteria* in paraffin oil. Without this adjuvant, which he referred to as the immunologists "dirty little secret," there is very limited protective immunity. Janeway proposed that there were specific receptors that recognized and responded to molecules present in the adjuvant and that this recognition event ultimately enabled T and B cells to produce a protective immune response. As such, the concept of pattern recognition and innate immunity, as we now know it, was born.

At the simplistic level Janeway proposed that infection was not recognized by the antigen receptors present on B and T cells, but by specific receptors on antigen-presenting cells (APCs), which were then able to provide the antigenic stimulus and costimulatory signals necessary to lead to activation of the B and T cells. He suggested that these receptors recognized highly conserved structures found in specific microbial products giving rise to the concept of a pathogen-associated molecular pattern, or PAMP. Adjuvants, therefore, must work by providing an appropriate stimulus for one of these receptors and as such "trick" the immune system into generating a protective response against the accompanying ligand (Fig. 1.3). The concept of PAMP-driven activation of the immune system also provided a rationalization for the ability of the host to differentiate between self and nonself molecules and stimuli. The race was then on to discover the identity of these so-called pattern recognition receptors, or PRRs, to elucidate the molecular basis of their functionality, and characterize the signaling pathways that they activate.

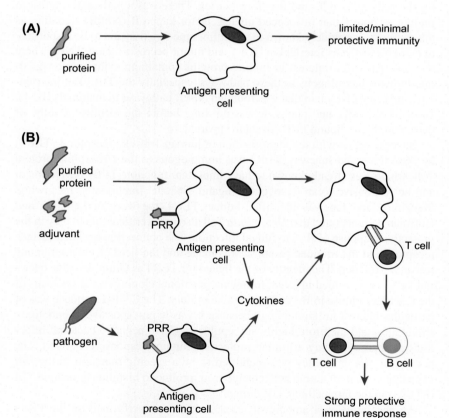

FIGURE 1.3   The detection of infectious nonself. Schematic overview of the theory put forward by Charles Janeway in 1989 that surface receptors, pattern recognition receptors (PRRs), were crucial for the recognition of immune stimuli and the initiation of protective immunity. (A) In the absence of PRR stimulation, only limited, if any, protective immunity is generated. (B) PRR stimulation in response to the presence of an adjuvant or a pathogen leads to cytokine secretion and enables antigen-presenting cells to present antigen, and provides helper and costimulatory functions to ensure that T cells and B cells can be activated to provide a strong level of protective adaptive immunity.

Early successes identified cell-free soluble receptors including cluster of differentiation 14 (CD14), which is involved in the detection of lipopolysaccharide (LPS) (see Section 4.1), and mannose-binding lectin (MBL), which is important in the activation of one of the three complement cascades (see Section 3.4.3). However, the cell-free nature of these receptors showed that they were not strong candidates for Janeway's hypothesis as they would only possess a limited, if any, capacity to modulate gene expression and therefore influence the development of protective immunity. Consequently a number of groups, including Janeway's own laboratory, focused their efforts on receptors in the membranes of macrophages and dendritic cells, the two types of APC important for the activation of T- and B-cell responses. There was a particular interest in finding receptors that influenced nuclear factor kappa B (NFκB) signaling as this pathway was widely known to affect immune function and to be responsive to cytokines such as interleukin (IL)-1 and tumor necrosis factor (TNF). There was also particular interest in finding proteins containing cytoplasmic signaling domains homologous to these pathways, especially the TIR (Toll/interleukin-1 resistance) domain that was found in NFκB pathways in mammals (IL-1), *Drosophila* (Toll), and plants. It was not long before the identity of some of these membrane-bound PRRs became apparent.

Success began with the identification of human Toll-like receptor 4 (TLR4) by Medzhitov and Janeway. TLR4 was homologous to the *Drosophila* protein Toll, which was already known to have important functions in fly development and be responsive to an endogenous ligand, Spätzle. Importantly, meanwhile Medzhitov and Janeway identified human TLR4, the work of Lemaitre and Hoffman demonstrated that *Drosophila* Toll also had a critical role to play in the protective response of flies to fungal infection. The connection between surface receptors and the immune response was made and the field of innate immune research exploded. The identity of the ligand for TLR4 as Gram-negative bacterial LPS was provided in 1998, following positional cloning of the *lps* locus of the C3H/HeJ mouse in Bruce Beutler's laboratory. The C3H/HeJ mouse was of particular interest in immunology because it was hyporesponsive to endotoxin stimulation and therefore highly susceptible to Gram-negative bacterial infections as there was only a limited protective immune response generated. The reason for this deficiency was identified to be a specific mutation in the *tlr4* gene that caused an amino acid change from proline to histidine at residue 714 (P714H) in the intracellular TIR domain.

An absolutely vast amount of research has been performed on the PRRs since their initial discovery, and this has led to relatively rapid discovery and functional characterization of a wide range of PRRs and involved thousands of scientists across the globe. In 2011 the Nobel Prize for Physiology and Medicine was awarded jointly to Jules Hoffman and Bruce Beutler "for their discoveries concerning the activation of innate immunity" along with Ralph Steinman for his "discovery of the dendritic cell and its work in adaptive immunity." As research on PRRs progressed, it became apparent that other families of PRR existed, in addition to the TLRs and the soluble receptors already recognized. These included cytoplasmic nucleic acid sensors such as retinoic acid–inducible gene I (RIG-I), inflammasome-forming proteins and other members of the nucleotide-binding, leucine-rich repeat (LRR)–containing receptor (NLR) family, and members of the C-type lectin (CTL) receptor family. The functions and mechanism of actions of these receptors have been discussed in much greater detail in Sections 2 and 4 in particular, whereas Section 5 discusses their association with the adaptive response in more detail and Section 6 introduces some of the major diseases associated with PRRs and other aspects of the innate immune response.

1.1.2 Self, Nonself, and the "Danger" Hypothesis

It is crucially important that the immune system is able to accurately identify potential sources of harm. Without this ability, organisms run a parallel set of risks. Firstly, they fail to mount an appropriate protective response to the threat posed by microorganisms and the host therefore rapidly succumbs to infection. Secondly, they inappropriately mount an unnecessary immune response to molecules of self-origin and consequently attack, damage, and destroy the host's own tissues and cells. Broadly speaking, the immune response is highly proficient in ensuring that these risks are not played out, but it is not infallible. Some pathogens do indeed successfully evade and subvert the immune response, and on occasion the immune response will inappropriately target host material, such as with the production of autoantibodies in autoimmune conditions such as lupus erythematosus.

During the latter half of the 20th century, the functionality of the immune response was explained by the self–nonself hypothesis. At its simplest the self–nonself theory states that the immune system learns to differentiate self as things encountered very early in life and nonself as things encountered later on. This was based upon the work of Burnet and Medewar and recognized the ability of lymphocytes (T and B cells) to recognize and respond to specific foreign antigens and that "self-reactive" lymphocytes were deleted early in life. As such the host becomes tolerant to self tissues, cells, and molecules, but intolerant to nonself molecules derived from exogenous sources and would consequently mount a protective immune response against these nonself components.

As our understanding of the mechanics of the immune response improved, changes were gradually made to the self–nonself hypothesis to account for observations that could not be easily explained by the original theory. These include the fact that the host organism is a dynamic entity and hence the concept of "self" changes with time, such as through puberty, pregnancy, lactation, and tumorogenesis. However, these events do not lead to wholesale immune attack. Similarly, the presence of the commensal microflora does not result in a continual immune response to try and remove these microorganisms. However, of course, if they cause damage to the host, they do become an immune target. In addition, as highlighted before protective immunity is only weakly, or not at all, generated in response to foreign material such as purified proteins that lack a suitable adjuvant.

Janeway's proposal that specific receptors, the PRRs, on APCs recognized conserved PAMPs on pathogenic microorganisms, provided a degree of rationalization of how self and nonself could be discriminated. Specifically, PRRs only recognized nonself, and only after recognizing nonself, were they able to provide the costimulatory signals that had been shown to be necessary for the activation of lymphocytes. However, regardless of how elegant and insightful his proposal was, it still does not fully explain the ability and range of self and nonself discrimination. For example, why do some microorganisms not initiate an immune response, and why does the host initiate an inflammatory immune response under conditions of sterile and noninfectious injury?

A further theory to explain immune specificity was provided by Polly Matzinger who put forward the "danger" hypothesis. In this she advocated that the source of the material recognized by PRRs did not matter and did not need to be from an infectious agent. She stated that it was the potential danger of the molecule to the host that was important and that therefore they could be either exogenous, i.e., pathogen-derived, or endogenous, i.e., host-derived, in source (Fig. 1.4). Consequently, the immune response would not be activated by harmless exogenous material, but would, however, be switched on by potentially harmful endogenous products. This would then allow the host to respond appropriately to all potential threats and also fits with the broad principles underlying the self versus nonself theory. Support for the "danger" hypothesis has been provided through the identification of various endogenous molecules such as ATP, cardiolipin, and mitochondrial DNA; and processes such as lysosomal rupture, mitochondrial damage, cell swelling, and nonapoptotic forms of cell death, which are all capable of initiating an innate immune response. More recently, there have been suggestions that we should consider the innate immune response as a tool that responds to damage rather than danger. As such the role of PRRs would be to recognize a range of exogenous PAMPs that indicate a high likelihood of damage occurring, along with a spectrum of endogenous danger/damage-associated molecular patterns (DAMPs), which signal that damage is occurring or has already occurred. The innate immune response can then be activated to begin the process of removing the threat and repairing any damage.

An ability to protect against cellular threat and danger is a universal property observable at the level of the simplest unicellular and the most complex multicellular organisms. Unicellular prokaryotes, for example, use restriction enzymes and clustered regularly interspaced palindromic repeats to protect against pathogenic threats. As cellular complexity has increased, we also see a gradual increase in the range and the complexity of the protective elements of the immune response. As Metchnikoff demonstrated, even the simplest multicellular organisms have cell types specific to phagocytic functions that appear

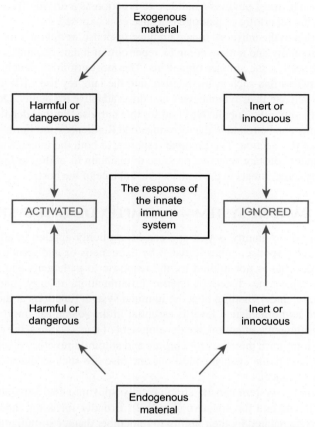

FIGURE 1.4   **The "danger" theory.** Diagrammatic representation of the principles of the "danger" theory of innate immune activation highlighting that the activation of the innate immune response is dependent on the threat presented by a molecule and not on whether it is exogenously or endogenously derived.

connected with immune defense—in unicellular amoebae, the engulfment of extracellular material, or phagocytosis, seems more directly related to the acquisition of food. The use of specific receptors on cell surfaces, i.e., PRRs, has been reported for a wide range of organisms of different evolutionary history and complexity. Interestingly the repertoire of PRRs shows some quite dramatic variation between different species and it is far from uncommon for there to be lineage specific expansions and losses of specific subsets of PRRs. For example, sea sponges have over 200 NLR and NLR-like receptors, whereas the Atlantic Cod has more than 200 TLRs. In contrast, humans have 22 NLRs and 10 TLRs. It is widely likely that these expansions and contractions are driven by environmental changes that influence the specific dangers these organisms are exposed to. The most obvious candidate to function as a driving force for these changes is the repertoire of pathogens a species is exposed to.

In addition to the universal innate immune response, vertebrates have evolved adaptive immunity and a more complex repertoire of innate responses to supplement those seen in the simpler organisms. The most primitive vertebrates composed of jawless fish such as the hagfish, and the lamprey use LRR–containing proteins to activate their lymphocytes and drive adaptive immunity. Other vertebrates use the immunoglobulin (Ig) fold for this purpose. Further details of adaptive immunity can be found in the recommended References and Further Reading at the end of this section. The immune response, at both the innate and adaptive levels, is under constant selective pressure to maintain its ability to fight off and neutralize specific threats to the homeostatic balance of the host.

1.2 THE IMMUNE SYSTEM—A COMPLEX DEFENSE SYSTEM

The concept of immunity is vast and can be explicitly applied to all forms of inflammatory response, either initiated by exogenous or endogenous sources. This includes, but is not limited to, the response to pathogens and microbial species, autoimmune disorders, sterile inflammation, allergy, and tumors. Consequently, understanding how the immune system functions at the molecular, cellular, and organismal level is essential in the search for improved treatments for pathogenic infection, the development of new vaccines, the generation of suitable long-term therapies for chronic and autoinflammatory disorders, and in the continual battle against conditions and diseases such as diabetes, atherosclerosis, and cancer.

The immune system can be simplistically split into two separate components, the innate and the adaptive (Fig. 1.2). Broadly speaking, these defense systems are segregated by their ability to remember danger stimuli and the type of response they initiate. In general the innate response, which in various forms is conserved across all multicellular organisms, is driven by germ line–encoded receptors that provide a response to danger signals derived from both internal and external sources. Regardless of the number of exposures to a specific stimulus, this results in the induction of a nonspecific generalized inflammatory response. As such, if all things are equal a repeat exposure to a specific immune stimulus will lead to a response identical to that initiated on the previous exposure.

The adaptive response in contrast appears to have developed only in vertebrates and provides specific long-term, sometimes lifelong, protection against pathogens. The adaptive response is characterized by the activation of T cells and induction of antibody production by B cells. The strength of the protection, which can be conferred by the adaptive immune response, is perhaps best exemplified through the success of the worldwide vaccination program that led to the global eradication of smallpox. Smallpox, spread by the *Variola* virus, was a highly contagious infection with high mortality rates.

Individuals were immunized with the less-virulent *Vaccinia* virus, a species closely related to both smallpox and cowpox. This led to the development of a protective adaptive immune response against the vaccine strain that provided sufficient cross-protection to render the individual immune to smallpox. This protection was lifelong and led to the global eradication of smallpox. The last reported case of naturally occurring smallpox infection was in Somalia in 1977. The only other known cases since then occurred in the following year, 1978, in Birmingham, United Kingdom and were due to accidental laboratory-acquired infection.

The adaptive and innate immune responses were originally believed to function independently of one another. However, it is now clear that they are, in fact, intrinsically linked. Indeed, activation of the innate immune response plays a crucial role in fine-tuning the development of the adaptive response, particularly in relation to the activation of particular types of T cell. This includes directing the differentiation of $CD4^+$ T cells into either T-helper (Th) 1, Th2, or Th17 subsets. In addition, the signaling pathways involved in immunity are multifaceted, highly complex, and heavily interconnected with a large element of cross talk. They also display strong evolutionary conservation. Consequently, almost all translational and animal models can, at some level, be applied to inform on immune function if analyzed in the appropriate manner. With closer scrutiny of the use of animals in research, we are seeing an expansion in the use of different species, such as zebrafish (*Danio rerio*), as models for immune function. With these, as with any model system, close attention must be paid to both the similarities and the differences in immune functionality, and it is not unheard-of for animal models to present in a phenotypically different manner to the equivalent condition in humans (see Sections 6.4 and 6.6).

The innate and the adaptive immune responses function over different timescales (Fig. 1.5). The innate response is in essence immediate. Recognition of a pathogen, the contents of a dying cell, or some other type of "foreign" material or "danger" signal, leads to the induction of a measurable physiological response within a matter of minutes. This response may take the form of the release of cytotoxic enzymes and chemicals from storage granules, the initiation of an acute phase response, the formation of macromolecular protein structures, and the activation of proinflammatory signaling. As we shall see through the rest of this book, there are many different manifestations and components to the innate response and these elements often work in an interconnected and regulated manner. Many of these responses such as cell death, the release of cytolytic enzymes, and reactive oxygen species (ROS) have the potential to be highly damaging to the host tissues and cells and are as such tightly regulated by control mechanisms that bring about the process of resolution and repair and help to restore the homeostatic balance. The extent of the innate response to immunological stimulation continues to rise for the first few hours after stimulation. Peak changes in gene expression are often observed between 6 and 24 h

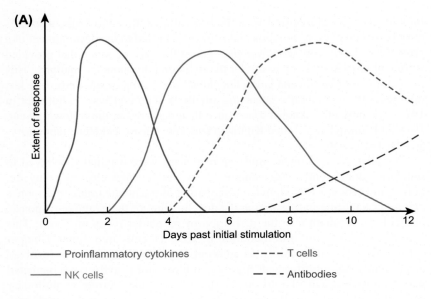

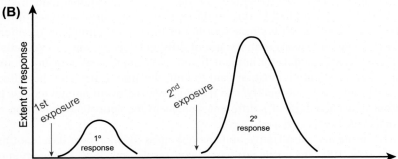

FIGURE 1.5 **The innate and adaptive arms of the immune response occur over different timescales.** (A) Graphical representation of the timepoints at which key components of the innate and adaptive immune responses are activated, peak, and return to baseline levels. Proinflammatory cytokine (red) production begins almost immediately, peaks around 2 days, and is over by 5 days. The natural killer (light blue) cell response begins around day 2, peaks around day 5–6, and tails off until day 11–12. T cell responses (*green dash*) begin around day 4 and peak around days 8–10. B-cell–mediated production of specific antibodies (*purple dash*) starts around 7–8 days and rises gradually. All times relate to number of days post the initial detection event. (B) Second exposure to an antigen results in stronger, more rapid response from the adaptive immune system.

poststimulation, depending on the specific genes involved. This often results in peak levels of cytokine secretion, an important class of immune effector molecule (see Section 3) within 1–2 days, which rapidly return to basal levels. In the case of viral infections the innate response from natural killer (NK) cells peaks slightly later around 3–4 days.

Activation of the adaptive immune response is a much more complicated process that involves multiple cell types, extensive intercell communication, wide-ranging and complex transcriptional and translational changes, and the induction of cellular proliferation. Consequently, it does not happen so quickly and can experience a delay of at least 3–5 days from stimulation with peak responses not beginning to occur until at least 7 days poststimulation. The adaptive response begins with the recognition of antigen, presented on APCs such as macrophages and dendritic cells, by T cells and B cells. This leads to the stimulation of T- and B-cell proliferation from a process known as clonal expansion. Differentiation of the T and B cells results in antibody secretion from B cells and direct killing by cytotoxic T cells. The T-cell response peaks first and the antibody titer gradually increases with time. The number of T and B cells will return toward prestimulation levels because of cell death via a controlled process known as apoptosis (see Section 3.5). However, some cells do not die but persist for long periods of time as "memory" cells.

As mentioned earlier the magnitude and nature of the innate response are identical upon restimulation with the same antigen. However, this is not the case with the adaptive response, which displays immunological memory. The first exposure creates a primary response, the next one a secondary response. The secondary response occurs faster and is stronger than the primary response as a result of the presence of "memory" cells that remember the antigen (Fig. 1.5). This can enable infections to be cleared even before they become symptomatic and is a key concept underpinning the success of vaccination (see Section 5).

1.3 FUNCTIONAL ELEMENTS ON THE INNATE IMMUNE RESPONSE

The innate immune response is wide-ranging and multifactorial. This is necessary to provide sufficient protective coverage against the broad spectrum of threats and dangers to which a host organism is exposed. Each of these components is in principle capable of contributing to or providing protection against all manner of threats. However, of course not all are always needed, and depending on the source of the threat, not all are always accessible. For example, respiratory pathogens cannot be countered by the hostile actions of stomach acid and bile salts. Broadly speaking, the immune system can be separated into four distinct categories namely: (1) barrier functions; (2) the immune tissues; (3) immune cells; and (4) protein and peptide defenses (Fig. 1.6). The major elements of each of these sections are briefly introduced below, and particularly in the case of immune cells and protein and peptide defenses are much more extensively considered in the later sections of the book. However, before we move on and discuss these four areas of the immune system, let us first consider inflammation.

Barrier Functions	Immune Tissues

• skin
• mucus
• acidity
• physical movement
• expulsion
	• primary
	  – bone marrow
	  – thymus
	
	• secondary
	  – spleen
	  – lymph nodes
	  – Peyer's patches
	  – mucosa-associated

Immune Cells	Proteins and Peptides

• granulocytes
• monocytes
• antigen presenting cells
  – macrophages
  – dendritic cells
 	
• lymphocytes
  – T and B cells
  – NK cells
	• pattern recognition receptors
	• complement
	• antimicrobial peptides
	• cytokines
	• chemokines

FIGURE 1.6   **The immune system has four main functional areas.** The immune responses are provided via four main functional areas: barrier functions; immune tissues; immune cells; and immune-functioning proteins and peptides.

Inflammation is possibly the clearest and most obvious manifestation of innate immune activation. In the 1st century BC, Celsus described the four cardinal elements of inflammation: *calor*, *dolor*, *rubor*, and *tumor*. These four descriptions correlate to heat, pain, redness, and swelling, respectively, and are all conditions that we can easily associate with. For example, imagine an infected spot, pimple, or cut at the surface of the skin. This area becomes swollen and raised; gains a deeper red color—coloration that can radiate outwards; is often warmer; and most definitely tender to the touch. These responses occur whenever an innate immune response is activated. They result predominantly from the recruitment of immune cells to the site of damage or infection, vasodilation, and the action of pyrogenic pathogen–derived molecules and cytokines such as IL-6. We should of course remember though that inflammation is a natural response aimed at protecting the host from greater harm and providing restorative functions to repair damage and restore a homeostatic balance. Acute inflammation typically lasts from a few hours to a few days depending on the cause. However, chronic inflammation can last for months, years, or even decades and, as we shall see in Section 6, underpins the pathogenesis of many diseases, including metabolic disorders such as diabetes, cardiovascular diseases such as atherosclerosis, arthritis-based diseases, and autoinflammatory disorders.

In many cases the elements of inflammation are localized and focused on the cause of innate immune activation. However, occasionally and particularly with infections, regardless of whether they themselves become systemic, these elements can become more widely activated. This is perhaps most obvious in the case of fever. The activation of PRRs leads to the production of proinflammatory cytokines. One of these, IL-6, migrates into the circulation and acts as a pyrogen—an inducer of fever. It does this predominantly through the activation of eicosanoid synthesis and signaling (see Section 3.4.2), working through the cyclooxygenase (COX)-2 pathway and stimulating production of prostaglandin (PG) E2. This induction of fever can itself stimulate an innate immune response and also activate the heat shock response (Section 1.5). Prolonged and excessive fever can be highly damaging, and even fatal, for the host; however, it should be remembered that thermal regulation is first and foremost a defense mechanism. Many pathogens are unable to replicate under increased temperatures and in the early 20th century fever therapy was often employed to treat bacterial infections such as syphilis. In these cases, fever was induced by infection with the parasite *Plasmodium* that causes malaria, which may of course not have been an optimal choice! The induction of fever is metabolically costly and in mammals it is estimated that an increase in core body temperature of 1–2°C requires an increase in metabolic rate of 10–20%.

1.3.1 Barrier Functions

The barrier functions of the innate immune system fall into two categories: physical barriers and chemical barriers (Fig. 1.6). These represent the true first line of defense against exogenous threats and dangers as they provide the first point of contact between the host and the danger. Indeed, if they are functioning properly, and are undamaged and unbroken, they provide an extremely effective protective system.

The most obvious physical barrier is the skin. It provides a "theoretically" impermeable layer of dead skin cells in the form of the epidermis. These are continually sloughed off serving to both block and remove microbes. Breaks in the skin can be a result of cuts, abrasions, wounds, injections, bites, and surgery, and provide an ideal route to bypass this protective barrier. The skin is also protected by the presence of secretions, such as sebum, which is formed from unsaturated fatty acids, and inhibits microbial growth. Other physical barriers are provided through the expulsive processes of urination, defecation, and vomiting, which all serve to flush away or expel pathogens. Of course, many gastrointestinal infections such as cholera, dysentery, and salmonellosis use these mechanisms to aid transmission.

Mucus membranes also provide a barrier function through the secretion of mucin, the formation of a protective mucus layer, and the physical trapping and blocking of microbes from cell surfaces. Visualization of the intestinal mucosal barrier highlights how effective this protective barrier is. Further protection is provided in the respiratory tract by the process of hair-mediated filtration and the movement of cilia on cell surfaces to capture and expel particles ad microorganisms.

Further innate protection is provided by additional chemical defenses. These include lysozyme—an antibacterial enzyme that cuts peptidoglycan in the bacterial cell wall—which is present in tears and saliva; acidic environments such as the skin surface (~pH 5.5) and the gastric juices of the stomach (pH 2–3); the presence of saliva to dilute microbial load and wash pathogens off the mouth's surface to be swallowed and destroyed by stomach acid; and the presence of compounds, such as hyaluronic acid, which impede microbial movement. Of course, some pathogens have evolved to evade and neutralize these defenses and even thrive in the niche environments created. For example, the bacteria *Helicobacter pylori* secrete enzymes to neutralize stomach acidity and enable bacterial growth.

1.3.2 Immune Tissues

The immune tissues can be broken down into the primary and secondary lymphoid organs. The primary lymphoid organs consist of the bone marrow and the thymus and are the locations in which the lymphocytes form and mature. B and T cells are both first produced in the bone marrow from their respective progenitor stem cells. B cells also undergo maturation in the bone marrow, whereas T cells migrate to the thymus and mature there. These two primary lymphoid organs are therefore acutely critical to the development of the adaptive immune response but play a less obvious role in the functionality of the innate immune system.

The secondary lymphoid organs are a more diverse range of tissues and cells. They include the spleen, a few hundred lymph nodes, the tonsils, Peyer's patches, and the mucosa-associated lymphoid tissue (MALT). They serve two major purposes. One is to act as a sight of activation of T and B cells and the other is to filter the blood, tissue fluid, and the lymph. The main sites of filtration are the spleen, for blood; the lymph nodes, for the lymph; and the MALT, for the tissue fluid. Lymph is a clear fluid found inside lymphatic vessels that has the same composition as the fluid around cells—the interstitial fluid. It therefore provides an accurate representation of the antigenic and cellular composition of these regions and serves to act as a delivery system for bringing antigens to the waiting T and B cells so that they can be activated following antigen presentation. It is therefore very important in the activation of the immune response.

Lymph is transported in the lymphatic vessels, where it is taken to the lymph nodes. Lymph nodes are small, bean- or pea-shaped structures that are usually not bigger than 2 cm in size and often measure less than a centimeter. Lymph enters the lymph nodes through the afferent lymphatics before exiting via the efferent lymphatics. While within the lymph node, microorganisms and dead and dying cells are filtered out and antigens that are present are internalized by APCs and used to activate T and B cells. Some APCs will also migrate from the tissues to the lymph nodes via the lymphatics. Recognition of the antigen stimulates cellular proliferation resulting in an increase in the number of cells in the lymph node. This causes the lymph node to increase in size and therefore a swelling of the lymph nodes is a very common symptom of infection and also of some cancers.

Lymph nodes function as antigenic sampling points and filtration devices for the lymph. Tissue fluid, however, is not filtered by highly defined lymphoid organs but by looser aggregates of lymphoid tissue, the MALT. MALT is found within the mucosal regions and is formed from small aggregates of T and B cells, which are often referred to as lymphoid follicles. Further details on the intestinal immune defenses and components of the MALT system can be found in Section 1.4.

Tonsils represent lymphoid tissue masses that are more structurally defined than the aggregates that make up most of the MALT but are less organized than lymph nodes. They do not serve a direct filtration role for the blood, the lymph, or the tissue fluid. They are, however, involved in the trapping of pathogens, particularly bacteria, and the presentation of associated antigens to macrophages for presentation to mainly B cells. The tonsils are located at the base of the tongue and in the walls of the nasopharynx and pharynx. Their surface is covered with invaginations that help to trap the pathogens. These trapped pathogens are then internalized via phagocytosis by the epithelial cells, which then transport the antigens and the bacteria to macrophages.

The largest of the secondary lymphoid organs in the body is the spleen. The functionality of the spleen is focused on the blood, or the systemic circulation, and it is particularly crucial for the generation of the adaptive immune response to blood-borne antigens, being the primary location for the activation of T and B cells. The spleen is formed from two morphologically distinct structures, the red pulp and the white pulp, which provide specific functions. The red pulp serves as a cellular filter for the blood and removes damaged, dying, and unwanted red blood cells. Coupled with this, it also acts as a molecular sieve and removes circulating chemicals and foreign material that may cause potential damage to the host. The white pulp is a center for immune cell activity and at any one time contains roughly a quarter of the entire lymphocyte population of the body. It is located around the arteries that bring blood into the spleen and efficiently removes antigens, including pathogens, from the blood to enable their presentation to the awaiting T and B cells.

1.3.3 Immune Cells

The innate immune response is heavily reliant on a wide repertoire of immune cells, each of which has specific functions. Within the circulatory system, cells can be broadly categorized as either red blood cells (erythrocytes) or white blood cells (leukocytes). Erythrocytes are small, highly abundant cells that make up the majority of the cells in the circulation. Leukocytes on the other hand encompass a broad range of cell types, which includes granulocytic neutrophils, monocytes and macrophages, dendritic cells, and of particular relevance to the adaptive immune system T and B lymphocytes. The different types of leukocyte have been briefly introduced in the following subsections and are described in more detail within Section 2.1.

In mammals, erythrocytes lose their nuclei during development and maturation. In humans, the half-life of a red blood cell is approximately 4 months, in amphibians this can extend to as long as 4 years. This additional longevity is likely to be related to the retention of the erythrocyte nucleus in the amphibian.

The primary function of erythrocytes is to facilitate gas exchange by the provision of oxygen and the removal of carbon dioxide. They also contribute to other homeostatic functions including the regulation of blood flow in skeletal muscle, the transport of sugars, maintenance of calcium and redox homeostasis, and the regulation of cellular proliferation. Erythrocytes that reach the end of their life or become senescent—cease to provide functional roles—are removed from the circulation by macrophages in the spleen and liver.

In a classical context, one does not associate erythrocytes with any particular involvement in the immune response. However, there is an increasing body of evidence connecting erythrocytes to a wide range of immune-related and antimicrobial functions. This repertoire appears to be more extensive in nonmammalian, and hence nucleated, erythrocytes. One of the most obvious associations is as a host for infection, and this is excellently demonstrated by the parasitic infection malaria, which is caused by infection of red blood cells with members of the species *Plasmodium*, such as *Plasmodium vivax* and *Plasmodium falciparum*.

The immune functions of the erythrocytes, despite their cellular abundance, have been relatively poorly studied. Red blood cells are known to play a role in the formation of immune complexes with bacteria, complement, and antibody; can create hemoglobin-derived peptides with antimicrobial properties; and may act as immune decoys. This latter function is provided by the expression of glycophorin-A on the surface of the erythrocyte, which has been proposed to bind to pathogen surfaces, sequester them, and thereby reduce the effective pathogen load. However, further research is needed to fully validate this theory. In nonmammalian vertebrates it is clear that erythrocytes express specific proteins designed to recognize pathogens and initiate an immune response. These include PRRs such as members of the TLR family (Section 2.2.4).

It is clear that erythrocytes have some role to play in the innate immune response to infection, with the specifics of this role depending to a degree on the species and the pathogen involved. However, it is clear that the most crucial cells involved in the innate immune response are found within the white blood cell, or leukocyte, populations.

1.3.3.1 Granulocytes

Granulocyte is the name given to a group of white blood cells that all possess multilobed nuclei, usually three lobes, and a significant number of cytoplasmic granules. The shape of their nucleus means that they are commonly referred to as polymorphonuclear leukocytes. This group of cells, composed of neutrophils, eosinophils, and mast cells, represents the most populous category of white blood cells, or leukocytes. Granulocytes, especially the neutrophils, one of the key cell types in the innate immune response and play an important role in the inflammatory process and early clearance of pathogens.

1.3.3.2 Monocytes

Monocytes are the largest of the leukocytes. They are found in all vertebrates and produced in the bone marrow before being released into the circulation. Under normal conditions, monocytes make up between 3% and 8% of the circulating cell population and their numbers increase in response to infection. The life span of a circulating monocyte is fairly brief and most undergo apoptosis after about 24h. Some monocytes do, however, migrate into tissues or to the sites of damage or infection where they subsequently mature into macrophages. In fact, monocytes are derived from the same common progenitor cell as macrophages and dendritic cells—the monocyte macrophage dendritic cell progenitor—and all three cell types have been categorized as part of the mononuclear phagocyte system first proposed by van Furth in 1968. In addition to their phagocytic ability, monocytes possess a range of internal and external PRRs that enable them to actively seek, destroy, and respond to pathogens and other dangers. A commonly used surface marker for categorizing monocytes is CD14 which, in conjunction with TLR4, is involved in the extracellular recognition of bacterial LPS (Section 4.1). Although over 90% of monocytes are usually positive for CD14 expression, there is actually a fairly large level of heterogeneity in the precise molecular expression profiles of circulating monocytes and numerous subpopulations have been described. It is likely that each of these distinct populations plays a niche role in the response to particular dangers, or to the exacerbation of chronic inflammatory conditions.

1.3.3.3 Antigen-Presenting Cells

APCs provide the key connection between the activation of the innate and the adaptive immune responses. The most important APCs are macrophages and dendritic cells, although other cells including neutrophils and B cells can also present antigen to T cells. Macrophages and dendritic cells possess a broad repertoire of membrane-bound and cytoplasmic PRRs and are key mediators of the innate response to damage through the secretion of various effector proteins, or cytokines (Section 3), which recruit other immune cells and shape the nature of both the innate and adaptive responses. They also serve to present antigen on MHC to T cells and provide suitable costimulation to enable the induction of adaptive immune responses (see Section 5 and References and Further Reading).

A key element of macrophage and dendritic cell function comes through the continual sampling of their external environment by macropinocytosis and phagocytosis. In most cells the process of macropinocytosis, the sampling of the external environment, is not a constitutive activity but can be induced by exposure to growth factors. In contrast, APCs such as macrophages and dendritic cells continuously perform macropinocytosis at exceptional rates. For example, it appears that in roughly 30 min, macrophages are able to internalize extracellular material that is equivalent to their entire cellular surface in quantity. Meanwhile, the capacity of dendritic cells to sample the external environment results in them "consuming" almost their entire volume in about 2 h. It is little wonder given these rates of sampling that the capture, processing, evaluation, detection, and presentation of antigen by these cells is such an efficient and sensitive process.

Macrophages are most commonly found in both the nonlymphoid and the lymphoid tissues (see Section 2.1), but can also be found in the circulation where they are likely to be derived from the differentiation of monocytes. In addition to their immune functions, macrophages play an important homeostatic role in the removal of dead and dying cells and the secretion of growth factors. Dendritic cells are derived from the common dendritic cell precursor in the bone marrow, which differentiate into predendritic cells that are then found in the circulation, the spleen, the bone marrow, and which migrate into the lymphatics and undergo maturation to conventional dendritic cells. Conventional dendritic cells migrate between tissues and tend to be fairly short-lived. They play an important role in the processing and presentation of antigens, particularly T cells, under homeostatic and inflammatory conditions. A second type of dendritic cell, the plasmacytoid dendritic cell, is found in the peripheral organs and the bone marrow. In addition to the presentation of antigen to T cells plasmacytoid dendritic cells are crucial cell types in the detection and response to viral infection through the production of exceptionally high levels of type I interferons (IFNs) upon viral detection. Plasmacytoid dendritic cells appear to have a longer life span than conventional dendritic cells. The key functions of macrophages and dendritic cells are discussed in Sections 2 and 5.

1.3.3.4 Lymphocytes and Natural Killer Cells

At the most basic level, lymphocytes can be split into two separate categories—B cells and T cells. These cells are the primary mediators of the adaptive immune response. Broadly, B cells are responsible for what is classically referred to as humoral (or antibody-based) immunity, while T cells drive cell-mediated immunity through cytotoxic (cell-killing) functions. The functional activation of B and T cells is heavily dependent on APCs such as macrophages and, particularly, dendritic cells. As we will see in Section 5, the direction and the balance of the adaptive B and T cell response is intrinsically linked to the innate response.

Our understanding of lymphocytes continues to develop. This development is strongly associated with ever-improving abilities to isolate individual cell types based on the presence, or absence, of particular surface markers or transcription factors. This has led to the identification of a subset of lymphocytes that contribute to the innate protective response and play an important role in the subsequent development and direction of adaptive immunity. These cells are known as innate lymphoid cells (ILCs). They are subdivided into specific lineages based on the repertoire of specific transcription factors expressed and cytokines secreted, in a manner analogous to classical T cells. Indeed some lines of thought suggest that ILCs may well be the innate immune responses equivalent to the T-cell subsets Th1, Th2, and Th17, which are very important for the adaptive response. ILCs appear to become enriched at mucosal surfaces in response to cellular insult or danger. The localized secretion of cytokines, in addition to the presence of other exogenous and endogenous soluble factors, drives the precise direction of ILC maturation and consequently influences how they contribute to the innate immune response, to immunopathology, and ultimately to the adaptive response.

Another form of lymphocyte, the conventional NK cell constitutes a critical component of the innate immune defense network and is an example of a lymphocyte with innate effector functions. There is now increasing evidence that a small subset of NK cells, traditionally viewed as short-lived cytotoxic effector cells, are in fact able to survive longer term and retain a degree of immune memory. NK cells make up around 15% of the circulating lymphocyte population and they are particularly important in the immune responses against microbial, especially viral, infection and tumors, but it has become apparent that they also play roles in the immune responses that occur during pregnancy and as a result of stem-cell transplantation. It is therefore essential that a full understanding of NK biology develops. NK cells can be split into discrete populations. These include conventional, or splenic, NK cells that develop in the bone marrow and are released into the circulation; thymic NK cells; and tissue-resident NK cells that have been identified in multiple tissues, especially the liver. The dominant population, and by far the most heavily studied, is the conventional NK cell. These discrete NK cell populations can be separated by the specific range of surface markers and transcriptions factors that they express and respond to and their development is tightly controlled by the expression of cytokines such as IL-15. The presence of chemokine receptors such as CCR2 and CCR5 allows specific recruitment of NK cells to sites of infection and inflammation.

The activation and function of NK cells will be explored in more detail in Section 2.1.7.1. Briefly, they mediate their innate immune roles through the release of cytotoxic proteins and enzymes that stimulate target cell apoptosis or antibody-dependent cell-mediated cytotoxicity and through the secretion of cytokines such as TNF and IFNγ that promote the phagocytosis of target cells by neutrophils and macrophages. The extent to which an NK cell is activated depends on the repertoire of activatory and inhibitory signals received and their interaction with other immune cells and the inflammatory microenvironment. For example, type I IFNs, and IL-12, -15 and -18 all serve to enhance the extent of the NK response and increase their cytotoxic capability. Target cells are often identified through the absence of MHC expression on their surface, a change that commonly occurs with virally infected and tumor cells.

1.3.4 Protein and Peptide Defenses

Broadly speaking, this classification encapsulates all the proteins and small molecules involved in the immune defense at both the innate and adaptive levels. Consequently it covers a vast selection of detection and effector processes. These include protein receptors involved in immune detection and activation, cytokine and chemokine effectors, antibodies, cytotoxic granule contents, antimicrobial peptides (AMPs), and enzymatic cascades such as the complement and coagulation pathways. In many ways these components underpin the functional elements of the immune response. Therefore rather than trying to cover all of these in detail, I will introduce a few of the major concepts at this stage and expand the mechanistic and functional details in subsequent sections throughout the book.

1.3.4.1 Pattern Recognition

The principles of pattern recognition have been introduced in Sections 1.1.1 and 1.1.2 when discussing the theories of Janeway and Matzinger in relation to the identification of threats to the host. The idea of pattern recognition applies to both the innate and adaptive immune responses. In the adaptive response, T and B cells recognize the specific shape, or pattern, of peptides presented on MHC on the surface of APCs such as macrophages and dendritic cells. Recognition is followed by a series of receptor–coreceptor interactions, which activate the T and B cells leading to the activation of defense mechanisms such as cytotoxic T cell–mediated cell killing and the production and secretion of neutralizing antibodies. The specifics of this form of pattern recognition have been covered in exquisite depth in some of the suggested References and Further Reading at the end of this section.

In the innate immune response pattern recognition drives almost if not all of the immune functionality observed. Membrane-bound and soluble protein receptors identify a vast array of specific exogenous and endogenous molecules that signify the presence of infection and/or the potential for damage to occur to the host. Pattern recognition forms the basis of the inflammatory response, the activation of complement, and the initiation of blood coagulation. Specific PRRs come in all manner of shapes and sizes and include scavenger receptors, CTL receptors, TLRs, NLRs, and multiple different intracellular nucleic acid sensors. Their activation invariably leads to the switching on of proinflammatory signaling cascades and the production of cytokines such as TNF, various interleukins and IFNs, which drive a protective inflammatory response. For example, the lipid A portion of bacterial LPS when released into the serum is bound by LPS-binding protein, which either neutralizes the potentially harmful effects of LPS, or ultimately leads to proinflammatory signaling via TLR4 and the production of inflammatory genes under the control of transcription factors that include NFκB (see Section 4.1). The process of pattern recognition and how it mediates immune responses is the primary focus of this book and is discussed in more detail in later sections.

1.3.4.2 Complement

The complement system is a long-standing and crucial component of the innate immune system that involves over 30 membrane-bound and soluble proteins. Its origins can be traced back to phyla as evolutionary ancient as the sea urchin. The action of complement was first reported in the 19th century through the work of Buchner and colleagues, who described a heat-labile component of blood that showed bactericidal activity. Further work by researchers such as Jules Bordet and Paul Erlich built on these early observations and developed various, at times competing, theories regarding the combined action of this heat-labile component, which we now know as complement, and heat-stable components (which later turned out to be antibodies) from the blood in killing pathogens. Gradually a fuller picture of the complexity of the complement system was developed as the range of protein components and their precise roles and relationships to one another became apparent. It is now clear that the complement system serves a broad protective function to the host and contributes to a wide variety of defensive and immune-related functions.

At the basic level the broad functions of the complement system can be split into three areas: (1) the activation of inflammation; (2) the opsonization (labeling) of pathogens and cells for clearance/destruction; (3) the direct killing of target cells/microbes by lysis. Looking at these areas in more detail and considering some of the wider roles of complement show that the complement system has crucial functions to play in: the detection, recognition, and ultimate clearance or destruction of pathogens and foreign antigens; the clearance of apoptotic cells and their debris; stimulating phagocytosis by identifying and labeling targets through opsonization; transporting, modifying and clearing antigen–antibody immune complexes; influencing and modulating the nature of cell-mediated immune responses; and promoting specific adaptive immune responses. There is also a darker side to the complement system. Inappropriately activated or insufficiently regulated complement can damage host tissues and cells, a process that can be enhanced by the action of autoantibodies that recognize self components of the host. The complement system has also been associated with the development of a number of rare autoinflammatory and autoimmune diseases that result from inappropriate or excessive activation of complement. These include neuromyelitis optica, atypical hemolytic uremic syndrome, and paroxysmal nocturnal hemoglobinuria. These conditions are often the result of rare genetic polymorphisms and their low rate of occurrence highlights the importance of complement, in that mutations in components of the complement system are not likely to be often compatible with long-term survival of the organism.

The complement system can be split into three separate enzymatic cascade pathways—the alternative, the lectin, and the classical—which are activated in this order and all converge on the production of a key complex known as the C3 convertase (Fig. 1.7). I will discuss these pathways in more detail in Section 3.4.3, and in Section 5. I will address the connectivity that the complement system provides between the innate and adaptive arms of the immune response.

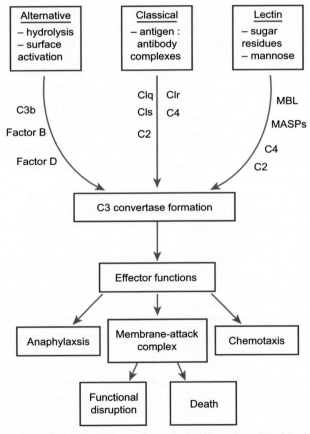

FIGURE 1.7 **The complement system.** A highly simplified representation of the three main activation cascades of the complement system, which converge on the production of a multiprotein complex that can function as a C3 convertase. The alternative pathway is presented on the left hand side, the classical pathway in the middle, and the lectin pathway on the right hand side. The identity of the C3 convertase, C4b2a, is shared for the classical and lectin pathway; but it differs for the alternative pathway where it is C3bBb.

1.3.4.3 Cytokines

A cytokine is the name given to a small protein, normally in the size range of 5–20 kDa, which is secreted from a cell in response to some form of stimuli. They are signaling molecules as they serve to induce responses from other cells. This intercellular signaling results from the interaction of the cytokine with specific receptors present on the surface of the target cell. Example interactions include those between TNFα and the TNF receptor, and IL-8 and its receptor C-X-C motif chemokine receptor 2. Depending on the exact cytokine involved, they are able to function on the same cell that secreted them (autocrine signaling), on neighboring cells (paracrine signaling), or on more distant cells in a systemic manner (endocrine signaling). Although the mechanism of action of cytokines is not that dissimilar to that of hormones, they are viewed as a distinct class of biological molecule. This may partly be due to the broader range of cells that are able to secrete cytokines. Cytokines display a wide range of functional diversity and this affects their broad classification. Among their many roles, they can also act as: stimulators of cell growth (e.g., platelet-derived growth factor and epidermal growth factor); proinflammatory mediators (e.g., TNF, IL-1); antiinflammatory mediators (IL-4, IL-10, TGF-β); and chemoattractant molecules (chemokines) to recruit immune cells to the site of infection, inflammation, or damage. Excessive cytokine production can lead to the creation of a "cytokine storm" and the induction of sepsis, which is hard to effectively treat and is associated with high levels of mortality. A more detailed overview of the major cytokines involved in the innate immune response has been provided in Section 3.

1.3.5 Cell Death

The process of cell death is an integral and natural part of the survival of an organism. Cell death is crucial to ensure the correct formation of tissues and limbs during the development of an organism. It is also essential to maintain homeostatic balance as it enables nonfunctional, old, worn-out, senescent, and unneeded cells to be disposed off, thereby minimizing the impact and metabolic cost of maintaining these cells. These cells can then be replaced by new cells produced in response to the specific needs of the organism. Cell death is also a key component of the protective response to infection and tissue damage. A dead cell cannot function as a host for microbial replication and hence many infections, particularly viral ones which are always intracellular, result in cell death.

Cell death can occur either in a controlled or uncontrolled manner. Initially, cell death was described as either being the result of apoptosis (controlled) or necrosis (uncontrolled). Apoptosis can be initiated by internal stimuli such as the release of cytochrome c from damaged mitochondria, or by external stimuli such as FasL or TNFα. These routes are known as the intrinsic and extrinsic pathways, respectively. A key difference between cell death via apoptosis and necrosis is that in apoptosis the cell does not release its contents into the extracellular milieu and therefore this does not cause damage to the surrounding tissues. In contrast, necrosis results in large-scale release of cellular contents including highly damaging components such as ROS and a range of lytic and digestive enzymes. These cause extensive damage to surrounding tissues and lead to further cell death and inflammation.

The process of initiating and facilitating cell death is, however, somewhat more complex than can be explained by simply categorizing it as being the result of either apoptosis or necrosis. For example, in addition to pathogen-induced cell lysis, which is very similar to necrosis, there are other mechanisms of cell death such as pyroptosis and necroptosis. Pyroptosis is driven by the activation of inflammatory caspases, whereas necroptosis describes the deliberate controlled induction of necrosis and commonly involves signaling pathways centered on the proteins receptor-interacting serine/threonine protein kinase 1 (RIPK1) and RIPK3. A more detailed description of apoptosis, necrosis, necroptosis, and pyroptosis has been given in Section 3.5.

1.4 THE MUCOSA-ASSOCIATED INNATE IMMUNE SYSTEM

There are four main surfaces at which the internal environment can come into contact with potential external threats. These are the bronchorespiratory tract, the nasopharyngeal tract, the urogenital tract, and the gastrointestinal tract. Each of these locations is exposed to its own particular repertoire of commensal and pathogenic microorganisms. By far the largest surface, both in terms of its size and also the range and variety of microorganisms it comes into contact with, is the gastrointestinal tract. The immune processes that function at these surfaces are often referred to as the mucosa-associated immune system, or MALT. Here I will focus on the immune defenses associated with the gastrointestinal tract. This reflects both its size and importance, but also that the majority of our understanding of how mucosal immunity works stems from research done on the gastrointestinal tract.

The gastrointestinal tract can be separated into three primary regions: the stomach, the small intestine, and the large intestine. The innate immune functionality of the stomach is straightforward and almost entirely dependent on the harshly acidic environment. However, some bacteria such as the cancer-causing *H. pylori* are still able to colonize the stomach as they possess a range of virulence factors that serve to neutralize the local acidic environment.

The function and physiology of the small and large intestine are distinct from one another. The primary role of the small intestine is to absorb nutrients ingested directly as part of the diet, or which result from microbiota-driven metabolism of dietary content. This latter group includes short-chained fatty acids such as butyrate that commensal bacteria produce upon the metabolism of dietary components such as fiber. Butyrate itself is an important modulator of immune function and also a key source of energy for intestinal epithelial cells. In contrast the major duty of the large intestine is to regulate absorption of water. Microbiologically the range and repertoire of bacteria is much greater in the small intestine in comparison to the large intestine. These factors all contribute to differences in the immune functionality at both the innate and adaptive levels in these two regions.

At the basic level the surfaces of the small and large intestine consist of a single layer of mucus-covered intestinal epithelial cells. This barrier serves to keep the contents of the intestinal lumen separate from the underlying tissues. Interspersed within, and below, the intestinal epithelia are a variety of cell types that provide immune functionality. By ensuring separation of the commensal microbiota and the underlying cells, this arrangement helps to limit unwanted and unnecessary inflammatory responses, but ensures that rapid activation can occur in response to perturbations and breaches of the protective barrier.

1.4.1 The Cells of the Gastrointestinal Tract Epithelium and Their Role in Innate Defense Mechanisms

The mucosal layer is formed from mucus secreted by goblet cells. Goblet cells make up around 15% of the large intestine's epithelial surface and provide a continuous, renewing source of mucus. The mucus layer can be split into two halves: an upper half that contacts the host microbiota and in which individual bacteria are often found and a lower half that, under normal physiological conditions, is free of microorganisms and provides an effective protective surface on top of the epithelium.

The majority of the epithelium in both the small and large intestine is made up of intestinal epithelial cells or enterocytes. These cells are derived from multipotent stem cells in the intestinal crypts. In addition to providing a physical barrier and absorbing nutrients from the lumen, the intestinal epithelial cells also have an important role in the detection of potential danger from microorganisms. These epithelial cells express a range of PRRs on their surfaces and also internally, including members of the TLR and NLR families. They are therefore able to identify and respond to the inappropriate presence of microorganisms that have managed to breach or traverse the mucosal layer and make contact with the epithelial surface. Expression of PRRs by intestinal epithelial cells is tightly regulated, reflects the most likely pathogens to be encountered, and is done in a manner to limit the unnecessary, or inappropriate, activation of an inflammatory response. For example, TLR5, which responds to bacterial flagellin (see Section 4.3.4), is only expressed on the basolateral surface of the epithelial cells. Consequently, it only becomes activated when the integrity of the epithelium is actually breached and bacteria are able to penetrate between or under the epithelial cells. Similarly, intestinal epithelial cells appear to have high levels of constitutive expression of NLRC4. This facilitates extremely rapid protective responses to bacterial pathogens seeking to invade or colonize the intestinal epithelial layer.

The intestinal epithelium also contains intraepithelial lymphocytes. These are mainly T cells that can be activated to secrete a variety of inflammatory cytokines. Lymphocytes, including ILC3 cells, are also found below the epithelium in a region known as the lamina propria. B and T cells in the lamina propria are able to be rapidly activated by APCs (macrophages, dendritic cells) that have received antigen either as a result of direct sampling of the luminal space following insertion of projections between epithelial cells or through the receipt of antigen translocated from the luminal surface via microfold (M) cells. It may well be that a large proportion of these intestinal antigens are transferred as cargos of endogenously formed calcium phosphate nanoparticles. These nanoparticles encapsulate the antigens and ensure they are trafficked through the M cells to the underlying APCs.

1.4.2 Peyer's Patches and M Cells

Peyer's patches are only found in the small intestine. They contain a T cell–rich zone, a germinal center for the activation and maturation of B cells, and a subepithelial dome rich in dendritic cells. Peyer's patches are the primary component of the gut-associated lymphoid tissue (GALT), which is itself part of the MALT. They are maintained in a manner broadly separate from the systemic lymphocytes. Peyer's patches are commonly associated with M cells. M cells are a specialized type of epithelial cell that has evolved specific functions to enhance the uptake of antigens from the intestinal lumen. Antigens coming through M cells are brought directly to APCs, often dendritic cells, in the Peyer's patch. In germ-free mice, their Peyer's patches do not develop properly, are smaller, and less numerous. This is likely to be a result of the loss of antigenic stimuli coming through the M cells and the subsequent reduction in lymphocyte stimulation, activation, and proliferation. The APCs are able to activate B and T cells in the surrounding Peyer's patch and also on occasion migrate to the draining lymphatics and travel to lymph nodes.

1.4.3 Secreted Defenses

The intestinal innate immune system makes extensive use of secreted defenses to protect itself from damage. Mucus secreted from goblet cells functions as a secreted barrier defense. Other active secreted defenses are also present in the form of AMPs and the antibody IgA. These molecules damage, neutralize, or destroy microorganisms that represent a threat to the host.

1.4.3.1 Antimicrobial Peptides

AMPs can be considered to be one of the most critical sets of innate immune defenses employed by a host. AMPs are used as effective defenses in potentially all eukaryotic organisms and for some organisms represent one of, if not all, the primary innate defense mechanisms. For example, some frogs secrete over 300

AMPs through their skin. AMPs can provide protection against the whole repertoire of infectious organisms—bacteria, fungi, parasites, and viruses. They are also produced by many prokaryotes. AMPs may be constitutively expressed by cells, or induced upon detection of danger, and in most cases the primary sites of AMP production are the epithelial surfaces because these are the most likely to come into direct contact with pathogenic threats.

AMPs are formed from peptide chains of at least five amino acids. While in theory there is no upper size limit to the peptide chain, in practice they are usually very, or relatively, short and rarely form globular structures. Most AMPs are cationic in nature, which helps recruitment to the negatively charged target membranes. However, a small number of anionic AMPs, such as dermcidin that is secreted from human sweat glands, have been reported. AMPs do not kill through enzymatic mechanisms. Hence, important antimicrobial proteins such as lysozyme, which kill bacteria through enzymatic cleavage of the bacterial cell wall component peptidoglycan, and secreted phospholipase A_2, which hydrolyzes bacterial phospholipids to disrupt membrane integrity, are not classified as AMPs.

The diversity and range of AMPs are readily apparent. At the time of writing, the publically accessible Antimicrobial Peptide Database holds records for 2718 AMPs across six different kingdoms and nearly 400 AMP structures have been solved. AMPs are normally classified into groups based on their structure. A number of different groupings exist but they commonly include: (1) alpha-helical; (2) beta sheet; (3) mixed structure; and (4) extended. The majority of AMPs are classified as either alpha-helical or as beta sheet. Examples of these structures have been shown in Fig. 1.8. In general, AMPs display an amphipathic character, i.e., they have a hydrophilic surface and a hydrophobic surface. AMPs can also be classified by their target—antibacterial, antiviral, antifungal, antiparasitic—or indeed by their mechanism of action as membrane active or intracellularly active.

As indicated earlier, most AMPs kill their target by either disrupting the membrane, for example, members of the cathelicidin and defensin AMP families, by interfering with essential intracellular processes such as RNA or DNA synthesis, or as in the case of β-defensin 3 disruption of bacterial cell wall synthesis. The cationic nature of almost all AMPs provides a strong charge-based attraction to the negatively charged target membrane and enables the hydrophilic portion of the AMP to interact with the head groups of the phospholipid bilayer. This is followed by the insertion of the hydrophobic part of the AMP into the hydrophobic fatty acid core of the membrane bilayer. This process either facilitates translocation of the AMP into the target or enables pore formation and target permeabilization and killing.

Some AMPs, particularly those that have antiviral activity, do not necessarily rely on direct killing as an effector mechanism, but instead may disrupt the interaction between the virus and the host cell; or induce changes in the host cell that lead to the creation of an antimicrobial (antiviral) state

nonpermissive for infection. For example, the AMP, NP-1 that was first isolated from rabbit neutrophils, protects against Herpes Simplex Virus type 2
infection by entering host cells and interfering with the nuclear migration of
the viral VP11 protein. This stops the virus from being able to initiate transcription of its immediate early genes and consequently causes a failure in the
establishment of infection.

AMPs can possess a broad spectrum of activity. This is beautifully demonstrated by indolicidin. Indocilidin is found in the granzyme secretions of bovine
neutrophils and it is active against bacteria, fungi, and viruses. Somewhat intrigu-
ingly its mechanism of action appears to be different against the different types
of pathogen. Fungi are killed as a result of direct damage to the cell membrane.
Bacteria are killed through a combination of approaches. Indolicidin is able to
cross the bacterial cell membrane and interfere with DNA synthesis; however,
much of its antibacterial activity has also been assigned to its ability to act as
an ionophore and shuttle negatively charged molecules across the membrane.
Meanwhile, its ability to target the virus HIV stems from an interference-based
mechanism in which indolicidin stops the HIV integrase protein from working and
therefore inhibits the insertion of the viral genetic material into the host genome.
Indolicidin itself is one of the smallest known AMPs consisting of just 13 amino
acids, over half of which are either proline or tryptophan. The full sequence is Ile-
Leu-Pro-Trp-Lys-Trp-Pro-Trp-Trp-Pro-Trp-Arg-Arg-NH2 (Fig. 1.8). Indolicidin

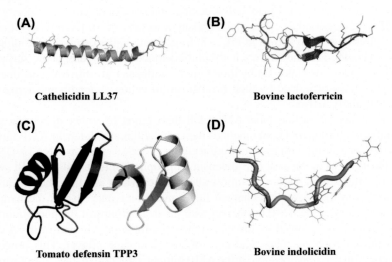

(A)

Cathelicidin LL37

(B)

Bovine lactoferricin

(C)

Tomato defensin TPP3

(D)

Bovine indolicidin

FIGURE 1.8 **Example structures of antimicrobial peptides.** (A) The alpha-helical antimicrobial peptide cathelicidin (PDB 2K60). Amino acid side chains are shown as lines. (B) The beta sheet
antimicrobial peptide bovine lactoferricin (PDB 1LFC), a derivative of lactoferrin. (C) The mixed
structured tomato defensin TPP3 (PDB 4UJ0) forms a dimer. (D) Indolicidin (PDB 1G89) has an
extended conformation without any definable secondary structure motifs when observed in the presence of dodecylphosphocholine micelles.

displays a degree of structural flexibility depending on the microenvironment, which is likely to reflect and contribute to the functional diversity displayed by this potent AMP.

Defensins are another family of AMPs that show broad activity against Gram-positive and Gram-negative bacteria, protozoan parasites, enveloped viruses and fungi. Defensins are small, though not as small as indolicidin, and generally range between 2 and 4 kDa in size. The formation of disulphide bonds between cysteine residues are critical for the formation of the overall structure adopted by defensins (Fig. 1.9) and hence underpin defensin function. Variations in the spacing between cysteines and the precise architecture of the disulphide bonds have led to the assignment of three major subgroups of defensin—α, β, and θ. Defensins are particularly important for protection of the gastrointestinal tract, which, because of its large surface area and the trillions of commensal bacteria that live there, presents a particularly challenging surface to protect.

Within the intestinal tract the different defensin subgroups appear to show cell-specific patterns of expression. α-defensins, such as HD5 and HD6, are only produced by Paneth cells; β-defensins–like hBD1 and hBD2 are secreted from epithelial cells throughout the small and large intestine; while θ-defensins, which are only found in Old World monkeys, are not expressed in the intestines at all but are instead secreted in the bone marrow and by leukocytes. Because AMPs, particularly those that target membranes, have the potential to damage host cells, their production must be tightly regulated. This can occur via a variety of mechanisms that include requirements for specific transcription factors, are dependent on PRR-mediated PAMP recognition, or involve posttranslational modifications that influence the relative affinity and toxicity of the AMPs for host and pathogen membranes.

Looking at the structure of α-defensins (Fig. 1.9), we observe a tendency for these molecules to pair together to form dimers or even, in some cases, multimeric filamentous assemblies. The human α-defensin HD6 is an example of a filament-forming AMP. As with many monomeric AMPs, the dimeric α-defensins are also amphipathic in nature, possessing a polar top surface and a nonpolar basal region. As described previously, this arrangement helps the AMPs to initially interact in a hydrophilic charge-based manner with the membrane surface, before inserting into the hydrophobic bilayer to create a pore or channel.

1.4.3.2 Immunoglobulin A

IgA is the second most abundant antibody in the serum after IgG and is the principal antibody secreted onto mucosal surfaces. The secreted form of IgA is usually referred to as sIgA. The vast quantities of sIgA produced mean that on a daily basis the host produces more IgA antibodies than it does of all other forms of antibody combined. The vast energy costs associated with such high levels of IgA, particularly sIgA, production highlight the critical importance it provides to the host as a defense against pathogenic infection.

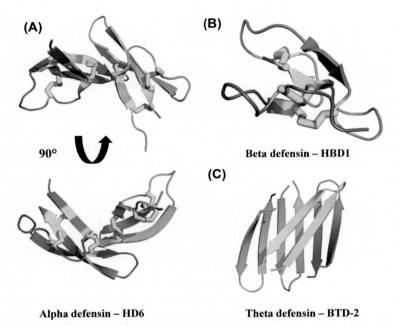

Alpha defensin – HD6   Theta defensin – BTD-2

FIGURE 1.9   **Example structures of alpha, beta and theta defensins.** (A) The alpha defensin HD6 (PDB 1zmq) forms a dimeric molecule. One chain is colored dark green, the other cyan. (B) The human beta defensin HBD1 (PDB 1KJ5) is found at high levels in urine and in breast milk. It exists as a monomeric protein. In panels (A) and (B) cysteine residues are colored yellow and the disulphide bonds they form are represented as *sticks*. (C) The baboon theta defensin BTD-2 (PDB 5inz) is a β-sheet antimicrobial peptide. The sheet is made of three BTD-2 molecules arranged in an antiparallel manner (cyan, green, pink). A fourth BTD-2 molecule (yellow) is placed on the top surface of the sheet. This fourth molecule is in an enantiomeric form different from that of the other three.

The structure of IgA follows that of all immunoglobulins (Fig. 1.10) and consists of a constant, Fc, region and two-variable, Fab, regions joined by a flexible hinge. These are formed from two identical heavy chains and two identical light chains (Fig. 1.10). Each of these chains adopts a classical Ig fold formed from a series of antiparallel beta sheets. The two isoforms of IgA, IgA1, and IgA2 that are expressed by humans show greatest variation in the hinge region, which is much larger in IgA1. It has been suggested that the difference in hinge dimensions may allow IgA1-derived IgA or sIgA to bind epitopes further apart on a target and hence have greater avidity for its target. It is the Fab region that is responsible for antigen recognition, and changes in the protein sequence at the tips of these structures enable recognition of a vast range of antigenic epitopes. The Fc region mediates interaction with receptor molecules that allow downstream signaling and cellular activation events to occur.

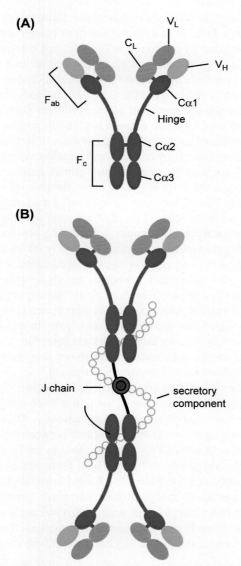

FIGURE 1.10 The structure of secretory immunoglobulin (Ig) A (sIgA). Schematic representation of the (A) monomeric and (B) dimeric forms of sIgA. Like all antibodies the molecule is composed of a constant (Fc) and a variable (Fab) region and contains heavy (V_H and $C\alpha1$-3) and light (V_L and C_L) chains. The likely position of the joining domain and the secretory component in the dimeric form is shown. Distinct domains are colored as follows: $C\alpha1$-3—dark blue; V_H—light green; C_L—tan; V_L—off-purple; J chain—brown; secretory component—light blue; and key disulfides between the Ig folds are represented by *solid blue lines*.

In the serum, IgA is found in a monomeric form, whereas sIgA tends to exist in a multimeric form, with dimeric molecules being most common. These dimers are held together by disulphide bridges formed between a small protein known as the J (joining) domain and the bottoms of the two Fc portions. This creates a broadly symmetrical molecule with a double-Y shape.

In humans, sIgA is produced in the GALT by antibody-secreting plasma B cells. Following its release from these plasma cells, the sIgA moves, in a polymeric form, toward the epithelium where it binds to the polymeric Ig receptor on the basolateral surface of epithelial cells at the mucosa surface. This stimulates endocytosis of the receptor:sIgA complex and vesicle-mediated transport to the apical surface. Cleavage of the receptor extracellular domain subsequently acts as a signal for the translocation of the sIgA into the mucosa in a complex containing the antibody and the secretory component of the receptor.

Following its secretion, some of the sIgA interacts with the commensal flora to help maintain homeostatic equilibrium. A major role, however, is in combating the effects of pathogenic microorganisms, particularly bacteria and their associated toxins. The protective function of sIgA is predominantly mediated through a process of "passive" neutralization whereby the sIgA molecules attach to the surface of the target and thereby inhibit its ability to bind target receptors, enter into target cells, or mediate toxic activity. The importance of sIgA is exemplified by the extremely high levels found in human colostrum and breast milk. Here sIgA provides a vital defense for the newborn against a wide range of pathogens. Indeed, numerous studies have conclusively shown that breastfeeding protects against both gastrointestinal and respiratory pathogens.

The importance of IgA as a host defense is further highlighted by the possession of IgA-targeting proteases by bacteria such as *Haemophilus influenzae*, *Neisseria meningitidis*, and *Streptococcus pneumoniae*. These bacterial proteases target the hinge region of the IgA1 molecule between proline and serine or proline and threonine residues. This cleavage releases the Fc portion of the IgA molecule and stops any ability to interact with Fc receptors on the surface of immune effector cells, thereby leading to a failure to initiate killing or clearance mechanisms. This evasion strategy is obviously much more relevant to serum IgA than to sIgA. Other streptococci, such as *Streptococcus pyogenes* and the highly pathogenic group B *streptococcus* secrete proteins that are able to bind and neutralize IgA molecules before they can interact with the pathogen surface.

1.4.3.3 Commensal Flora

The commensal flora relates to the microbial population living on the host organism and usually refers to the bacterial contribution. This is dominated by the intestinal microflora, but also includes contributions from other mucosal surfaces such as the urogenital and respiratory tracts, as well as patches of the skin. The numerical size of this bacterial population is vast and for humans it has long been stated that there are roughly 10 times as many bacterial cells on our bodies as cells of our own. For an average-sized human weighing around 70 kg, this would equate to around 30 trillion host cells and 300 trillion bacterial cells. However, this assumption has recently been challenged and in fact the number of bacterial cells may actually be roughly equal to the number of host cells. Interestingly, this number probably only contains in the order of 1000 different species. Regardless of the precise number present, there are an awful lot of bacterial cells present and they not only play a crucial role in digestion and nutrient acquisition, but also have an important and diverse role to play in immune defense and the regulation of both intestinal and systemic immune responses. For example they:

- inhibit pathogen growth by competing for space and nutrients and secreting compounds with antimicrobial properties,
- enhance the development and improve the efficiency with which immune effector cells such as neutrophils, NK cells, and Mast cells work,
- drive the production of sIgA,
- stimulate the proliferation of intestinal epithelial cells and their expression of antimicrobial genes, thereby helping to maintain protective barrier functions,
- induce the differentiation of CD4$^+$ T cells: *Clostridium spp* stimulate Treg development, segmented filamentous bacteria encourage Th17 cells, and the polysaccharide A component of *Bateriodes fragilis* promotes Th1 differentiation,
- repress the proinflammatory nature of the innate immune response, especially of intestinal macrophages, which is achieved through stimulating enhanced secretion of antiinflammatory IL-10, and by encouraging expression of SIGIRR (single Ig IL-1 receptor-related molecule) and PPARγ (peroxisome proliferators–activated receptor-γ), and
- germ-free animals show lower levels of sIgA, smaller and fewer Peyer's patches, reduced cytolytic activity of γδ T cells and reduced number and functionality of neutrophils and macrophages.

Given the numerous ways in which the commensal flora influences the immune response, it is not surprising that it has also been associated with the development and progression of various autoinflammatory and autoimmune diseases such as rheumatoid arthritis, inflammatory bowel disease (IBD), type 1 diabetes (T1D), and allergies. Consequently, changes in the composition of the microflora can have important health effects. The makeup of the microflora can show dramatic differences between individuals and is heavily influenced by diet, environment, and medications such as antibiotics. As the fetus is sterile before birth, the manner of delivery also influences the microbiota composition, most noticeably of the intestines. Babies delivered naturally are predominantly colonized by species of *Lactobacillus* and *Prevotella*, whereas those delivered by Caesarean section tend to be colonized by species of bacteria, such as *Staphylococcus, Corynebacterium*, and *Propionibacterium*, normally predominant on the skin. Early feeding methods also heavily influence the composition of the intestinal flora, which is likely to contribute to part of the high protection against intestinal infections provided by breastfeeding.

1.5 ADDITIONAL HOMEOSTATIC FUNCTIONS INVOLVED IN INNATE IMMUNE RESPONSES

1.5.1 The Heat Shock Response

The innate immune response responds to tissue insult and injury. One potential source of tissue damage is temperature. This could be excess cold resulting in a slow down in the rate of the cellular biochemistry or more radically the freezing and potential rupture of cells; or it could also be mild increases in temperature resulting in a loss of protein function due to protein unfolding or necrotic death due to extremely high temperatures as occurs with burns. Extreme temperature stresses cannot be immediately countered at the physiological level and so in the cases of temperature-induced cell death the innate response is crucially involved in clearing the damage and limiting the wider impact. In contrast, the cellular impact of temperature changes that do not lead to immediate cell death and may in fact only be a few degrees different to the optimal cellular temperature can be mitigated against by the induction of the heat shock response.

Small increases in temperature can result in protein aggregation and unfolding. As temperature increases, the cellular cytoskeletal network becomes disorganized and ultimately collapses leading to wide-scale cellular disorganization and an inability to move and transport molecules around the cell in an organized manner.

1.5.2 The Unfolded Protein Response

Correctly folded proteins are essential for correct cell function. High levels of unfolded or incorrectly folded proteins can induce intense metabolic, physiological, and functional stress upon the cell. This is most pronounced in the endoplasmic reticulum (ER). Unfolded proteins are also able to initiate an inflammatory response via activation of the unfolded protein response (UPR). The UPR is activated by three different protein sensors in the ER membrane. These are inositol-requiring enzyme 1 (IRE1), protein kinase R-like ER kinase (PERK), and activating transcription factor 6 (ATF6). Their activation leads to alterations in protein expression at both the transcriptional and translational levels with the aim of enabling the cell to restore homeostatic balance. These pathways interface with a range of inflammatory signaling cascades and lead to increases in the transcription of NFκB, stress kinase, and interferon-responsive genes. It has also been suggested that activation of TLRs can initiate the UPR as can certain NLR sensors including nucleotide oligomerization domain 1 (NOD1) and NOD2. The UPR may well contribute to the pathogenesis of some forms of IBD such as Crohn's Disease (see Section 6.5).

1.5.3 Autophagy

Autophagy is the process of self-eating. It is conserved across eukaryotes, represents an important mechanism in the maintenance of cellular homeostasis, and

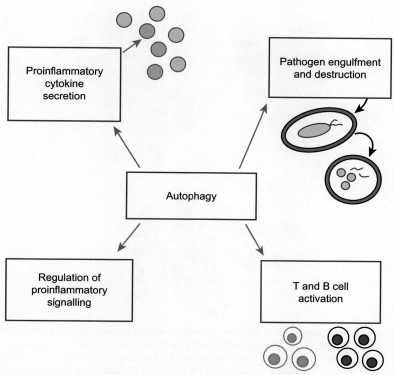

FIGURE 1.11   The link between autophagy and immune function. The process of autophagy is connected with a range of different innate and adaptive immune functions.

is being increasingly connected to immunological functions (Fig. 1.11). More specifically, autophagy involves the formation of double-membraned structures in the cytoplasm and is driven by a collection of proteins known as autophagy-related proteins (Fig. 1.12). At the homeostatic level, autophagy serves to enable the recycling of cytoplasmic contents to enable: (1) the breakdown of unwanted or dysfunctional organelles; (2) the reuse of macromolecules such as amino acids for structural or metabolic purposes; (3) the removal of large macromolecular aggregates; and (4) the regulation of cell death and cell-survival processes. From an immunological perspective, autophagy interfaces with both the innate and the adaptive arms of the immune system and contributes to: (1) the secretion of inflammatory and immune mediators and cytokines; (2) the engulfment and destruction of pathogens; (3) the regulation of proinflammatory signaling; and (4) the activation of T and B cells. Many of these pathways coincide and interface with PRR signaling, which is known to be able to activate autophagy and highlights the integrated nature of the innate defenses against infection, danger, and damage.

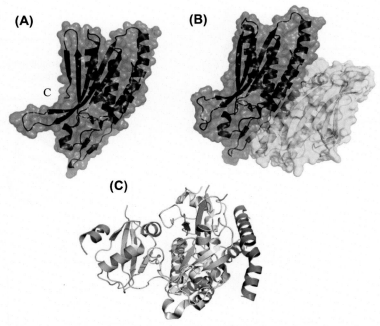

FIGURE 1.12 **Example structures of proteins involved in autophagy.** (A) The protein ATG101 (PDB 1WZG) is an essential component in the initiation of autophagy and adopts a protein fold known as a HORMA domain. The C-terminus of the protein is labeled. (B) Complex between ATG101 and the HORMA domain of ATG13 (PDB 5C50) that form part of the ULK complex along with ULK1 and FIP200, which initiates the process of autophagy. The ATG101 HORMA domain only experiences minor conformational changes upon binding. (C) A complex between ATG12 (salmon), ATG5 (gray), and fragments of ATG3 (orange) and ATG16L1 (blue). Image generated from PDB 4NAW.

REFERENCES AND FURTHER READING

Sections 1.1. and 1.2

Bretscher P, Cohn M. A theory of self-nonself discrimination: paralysis and induction involve the recognition of one and two determinants on an antigen, respectively. Science September 11, 1970;169(3950):1042–9.

Bretscher PA, Cohn M. Minimal model for the mechanism of antibody induction and paralysis by antigen. Nature November 2, 1968;220(5166):444–8.

Janeway CA. Approaching the asymptote? Evolution and revolution in immunology. Cold Spring Harb Symp Quant Biol January 1989;54(Pt 1):1–13.

Lederberg J. Genes and antibodies. Science June 19, 1959;129(3364):1649–53.

Lemaitre B, Nicolas E, Michaut L, Reichhart JM, Hoffmann JA. The dorsoventral regulatory gene cassette spätzle/Toll/cactus controls the potent antifungal response in Drosophila adults. Cell September 20, 1996;86(6):973–83.

Matzinger P. Tolerance, danger, and the extended family. Annu Rev Immunol 1994;12:991–1045.

Matzinger P. An innate sense of danger. Semin Immunol October 1998;10(5):399–415.

Matzinger P. Essay 1: the danger model in its historical context. Scand J Immunol 2001;54(1–2):4–9.

Matzinger P. The danger model: a renewed sense of self. Science April 12, 2002;296(5566):301–5.

Medzhitov R, Preston-Hurlburt P, Janeway Jr CA. A human homologue of the *Drosophila* Toll protein signals activation of adaptive immunity. Nature 1997;388(6640):394–7.

Medzhitov R, Janeway CA. Innate immunity: impact on the adaptive immune response. Curr Opin Immunol February 1997;9(1):4–9.

Medzhitov R. Approaching the asymptote: 20 years later. Immunity June 2009;30(6):766–75.

Merad M, Sathe P, Helft J, Miller J, Mortha A. The dendritic cell lineage: ontogeny and function of dendritic cells and their subsets in the steady state and the inflamed setting. Annu Rev Immunol March 21, 2013;31(1):563–604.

Murphy K, Weaver C. Janeway's Immunobiology. 9th ed. Garland Science Taylor & Francis Group; 2016. 928 pp.

O'Neill LAJ, Golenbock D, Bowie AG. The history of Toll-like receptors—redefining innate immunity. Nat Rev Immunol May 17, 2013;13(6):453–60.

Pancer Z, Cooper MD. The evolution of adaptive immunity. Annu Rev Immunol April 2006;24(1):497–518.

Peaper DR, Cresswell P. Regulation of MHC class I assembly and peptide binding. Annu Rev Cell Dev Biol November 2008;24(1):343–68.

Poltorak A, He X, Smirnova I, Liu MY, Van Huffel C, Du X, et al. Defective LPS signaling in C3H/HeJ and C57BL/10ScCr mice: mutations in *Tlr4* gene. Science December 11, 1998;282(5396):2085–8.

Pradeu T, Cooper EL. The danger theory: 20 years later. Front Immunol 2012;3.

Rossjohn J, Gras S, Miles JJ, Turner SJ, Godfrey DI, McCluskey J. T cell antigen receptor recognition of antigen-presenting molecules. Annu Rev Immunol March 21, 2015;33(1):169–200.

Stavnezer J, Guikema JEJ, Schrader CE. Mechanism and regulation of class switch recombination. Annu Rev Immunol April 2008;26(1):261–92.

Section 1.3

Casadevall A. Thermal restriction as an antimicrobial function of fever. PLoS Pathog May 5, 2016;12(5):e1005577. Hogan D.A., editor.

Evans SS, Repasky EA, Fisher DT. Fever and the thermal regulation of immunity: the immune system feels the heat. Nat Rev Immunol May 15, 2015;15(6):335–49.

Geissmann F, Manz MG, Jung S, Sieweke MH, Merad M, Ley K. Development of monocytes, macrophages, and dendritic cells. Science February 5, 2010;327(5966):656–61.

Junt T, Scandella E, Ludewig B. Form follows function: lymphoid tissue microarchitecture in antimicrobial immune defence. Nat Rev Immunol October 2008;8(10):764–75.

Pearson C, Uhlig HH, Powrie F. Lymphoid microenvironments and innate lymphoid cells in the gut. Trends Immunol June 2012;33(6):289–96.

Varol C, Mildner A, Jung S. Macrophages: development and tissue specialization. Annu Rev Immunol March 21, 2015;33(1):643–75.

Section 1.4

Bahar A, Ren D. Antimicrobial peptides. Pharmaceuticals November 28, 2013;6(12):1543–75.

Baxter AA, Richter V, Lay FT, Poon IKH, Adda CG, Veneer PK, et al. The tomato defensin TPP3 binds phosphatidylinositol (4,5)-bisphosphate via a conserved dimeric cationic grip conformation to mediate cell lysis. Mol Cell Biol June 1, 2015;35(11):1964–78.

Ignacio A, Morales CI, Câmara NOS, Almeida RR. Innate sensing of the gut microbiota: modulation of inflammatory and autoimmune diseases. Front Immunol February 19, 2016;7.

Mantis NJ, Rol N, Corthésy B. Secretory IgA's complex roles in immunity and mucosal homeostasis in the gut. Mucosal Immunol November 5, 2011;4(6):603–11.

Mcdermott AJ, Huffnagle GB. The microbiome and regulation of mucosal immunity. Immunology 2014;142(1):24–31.

Mukherjee S, Hooper LV. Antimicrobial defense of the intestine. Immunity January 2015;42(1):28–39.

Schibli DJ, Hunter HN, Aseyev V, Starner TD, Wiencek JM, McCray PB, et al. The solution structures of the human beta-defensins lead to a better understanding of the potent bactericidal activity of HBD3 against *Staphylococcus aureus*. J Biol Chem March 8, 2002;277(10):8279–89.

Szyk A, Wu Z, Tucker K, Yang D, Lu W, Lubkowski J. Crystal structures of human alpha-defensins HNP4, HD5, and HD6. Protein Sci December 2006;15(12):2749–60.

Wang G. Structures of human host defense cathelicidin LL-37 and its smallest antimicrobial peptide KR-12 in lipid micelles. J Biol Chem November 21, 2008;283(47):32637–43.

Wang CK, King GJ, Conibear AC, Ramos MC, Chaousis S, Henriques ST, et al. Mirror images of antimicrobial peptides provide reflections on their functions and amyloidogenic properties. J Am Chem Soc May 4, 2016;138(17):5706–13.

Section 1.5

Celli J, Tsolis RM. Bacteria, the endoplasmic reticulum and the unfolded protein response: friends or foes? Nat Rev Microbiol February 2015;13(2):71–82.

Colaço HG, Moita LF. Initiation of innate immune responses by surveillance of homeostasis perturbations. FEBS J July 2016;283(13):2448–57.

Deretic V. Autophagy as an innate immunity paradigm: expanding the scope and repertoire of pattern recognition receptors. Curr Opin Immunol February 2012;24(1):21–31. Elsevier Ltd.

Deretic V. Autophagy: an emerging immunological paradigm. J Immunol July 1, 2012;189(1):15–20.

Deretic V, Saitoh T, Akira S. Autophagy in infection, inflammation and immunity. Nat Rev Immunol September 25, 2013;13(10):722–37.

Janssens S, Pulendran B, Lambrecht BN. Emerging functions of the unfolded protein response in immunity. Nat Immunol September 18, 2014;15(10):910–9.

Levine B, Mizushima N, Virgin HW. Autophagy in immunity and inflammation. Nature January 20, 2011;469(7330):323–35.

Metlagel Z, Otomo C, Takaesu G, Otomo T. Structural basis of ATG3 recognition by the autophagic ubiquitin-like protein ATG12. Proc Natl Acad Sci USA November 19, 2013;110(47):18844–9.

Michel M, Schwarten M, Decker C, Nagel-Steger L, Willbold D, Weiergräber OH. The mammalian autophagy initiator complex contains 2 HORMA domain proteins. Autophagy 2015;11(12):2300–8.

Osterloh A, Breloer M. Heat shock proteins: linking danger and pathogen recognition. Med Microbiol Immunol March 2008;197(1):1–8.

Qi S, Kim DJ, Stjepanovic G, Hurley JH. Structure of the human Atg13-Atg101 HORMA heterodimer: an interaction hub within the ULK1 complex. Structure October 6, 2015;23(10):1848–57.

Sender R, Fuchs S, Milo R. Revised estimates for the number of human and bacteria cells in the body. PLoS Biol January 2016;14(8):e1002533.

Sumpter R, Levine B. Autophagy and innate immunity: triggering, targeting and tuning. Semin Cell Dev Biol September 2010;21(7):699–711.

Tanoue T, Umesaki Y, Honda K. Immune responses to gut microbiota-commensals and pathogens. Gut Microbes July 27, 2010;1(4):224–33.

Wu H-J, Wu E. The role of gut microbiota in immune homeostasis and autoimmunity. Gut Microbes January 27, 2012;3(1):4–14.

Zuo D, Subjeck J, Wang X-Y. Unfolding the role of large heat shock proteins: new insights and therapeutic implications. Front Immunol March 1, 2016;7.

Section 2

Immune Cells and the Process of Pattern Recognition

The innate immune system is far from simple. For it to function efficiently, it requires the integrated involvement of physical barriers, chemical defenses, enzymatic cascades, protein receptors, signaling molecules, and a host of different and diverse cell types. This section provides an overview of two key components of the innate immune system—the immune cells and the pattern recognition receptors or PRRs. It will introduce and summarize the roles of the key cell types involved in mediating a large proportion of the innate response. This includes cells such as macrophages and neutrophils, which possess well-described and obviously important roles in the detection and destruction of potential pathogen-based and endogenous dangers and threats. It also includes cells less commonly associated with the innate immune response, such as eosinophils and innate lymphocytes. The section will also describe the function of PRRs found at the cell surface and also within the cell. The importance of pattern recognition in the defense against both exogenous and endogenous dangers will become apparent. In a number of cases, later sections of the book will further develop and expand upon ideas and concepts introduced at this stage thereby allowing you to gradually build and enhance your understanding of innate immunity.

2.1 THE CELLULAR BASIS OF THE INNATE IMMUNE SYSTEM

All innate immune defenses involve cells in some form or other. This could be through the actual formation of physical barriers as occurs with skin cells and the intestinal epithelium; the secretion of chemical defenses such as antimicrobial peptides or hydrogen ions that contribute to stomach acidity; the secretion of mucus; the production and secretion of cytokines, chemokines, complement factors, eicosanoids, or other chemical mediators; or in the direct detection of danger. Here I will briefly describe the major elements of innate immune functionality for the major cell types involved most directly in the recognition and immediate response to danger.

The Innate Immune System. http://dx.doi.org/10.1016/B978-0-12-804464-3.00002-8

41

2.1.1 Monocytes

Monocytes play an important role in the response to infection and damage. Traditionally, circulating monocytes were believed to function as precursors of macrophages that were recruited to the sites of infection, damage, and inflammation, where they then underwent differentiation into macrophages. However, while monocytes can and clearly do differentiate into macrophages, the primary source of tissue-resident macrophages are macrophage progenitor cells placed into tissues during embryogenesis and prenatal development (see Section 2.1.2). This revised understanding of the relationship between monocytes and macrophages has led to reconsideration of the precise role of the monocyte in an immune and a nonimmune perspective. For example, do macrophages derived from embryonic progenitor cells differ from those derived from monocytes? Do monocytes have immune effector functions and what is their actual role in managing and mediating inflammatory responses and the process of resolution?

Monocytes are produced in the bone marrow from the common myeloid precursor through the process of hematopoiesis. This process is broadly controlled by macrophage-colony stimulating factor (M-CSF). Monocytes are released into the circulation and will undergo apoptosis and clearance within a day or two if not recruited to a tissue. These monocytes are not homogenous in nature, possess a variety of different surface markers, and can be classified on the basis of the presence or absence of markers such as CD14 and CD16. Different monocyte subsets have been proposed based on a combination of surface marker expression, location, and effector functions. Even without differentiating to macrophages, monocytes appear able to perform at least some immune effector functions. These include cytokine secretion, reactive oxygen species (ROS), and nitric oxide production and the killing of bacteria via phagocytosis. It has also been suggested that under certain circumstances, monocytes can help activate T cells. These processes are not, however, as efficient or potent as when performed by a macrophage.

Under homeostatic conditions, monocytes have a surveillance role in the detection of viruses and bacteria on the circulatory endothelium. Interestingly, they appear to use TLR7 as the primary PRR suggesting that viruses are the main pathogen of interest. In addition, upon PRR activation the inflammatory response appears to be initially tempered to allow clearance of the virus without additional damage to the vasculature. In inflammatory conditions, monocytes are recruited to the site of inflammation in response to the chemokines CCL2 and CX3CL1, where they help with the uptake of antigen and its presentation in lymph nodes, stimulate tissue repair, and differentiate into proinflammatory macrophages.

2.1.2 Macrophages

Macrophages, like monocytes, are immune cells of the myeloid lineage. They are members of the mononuclear phagocytic system and are derived from the monocyte macrophage dendritic common precursor. They are highly active in the process of phagocytosis; serve as a professional antigen-presenting cells (APCs) to facilitate activation of other immune cells; and play an important role in the removal of dead, dying, and damaged cells. They are an essential component in the development of the whole organism during which they actively phagocytose and remove cells that are no longer needed. This contributes to the functional organization of tissues and the correct development of complex structures such as limbs and digits. In addition to this developmental role, macrophages provide a crucial role in the detection and clearance of pathogens, maintenance of tissue homeostasis, and the induction, regulation and resolution of inflammation.

Macrophages can be separated into two distinct populations, those found in the circulatory system and those in tissues. These populations are often referred to as monocyte-derived macrophages and tissue-resident macrophages, respectively. For a long time, the general view held was that tissue-resident macrophages were the result of circulating monocytes migrating into the tissues upon the receipt of appropriate chemotactic signals, such as IL-8 or monocyte chemoattractant protein-1 (MCP-1), and then differentiating into macrophages in the tissues. However, more recently it has become clear that while monocytes do indeed migrate out of the circulation and differentiate into macrophages in tissues, primarily in response to infection and inflammation, this is not the source of the majority of tissue-resident macrophages. In fact it appears that most tissue-resident macrophages are actually integral components of the tissue and are deposited before birth, i.e., prenatally. The maintenance of this population is therefore reliant, not on hematopoiesis as occurs with monocyte-derived macrophages, but instead results from a combination of longevity and self-renewal.

It goes without saying that not all macrophages are phenotypically and functionally the same. A major difference occurs in the degree of proinflammatory character displayed by the macrophage. Monocyte-derived macrophages at the site of inflammation are generally highly proinflammatory in nature and are often referred to as M1 or classical macrophages. In contrast, macrophages with an antiinflammatory phenotype are often known as M2 macrophages. These M2 macrophages are more commonly derived from the tissue-resident macrophage population. M1 macrophages are formed when differentiation is stimulated by granulocyte-macrophage colony-stimulating factor (GM-CSF) and M2 macrophages predominate if this stimulation is provided by CSF-1. Their development is also promoted by the presence of proinflammatory (e.g., IFNγ, IL-1β, TNF) and antiinflammatory (e.g., IL-4, IL-10, TGF-β), respectively.

Somewhat unsurprisingly, tissue-resident macrophages in particular show functional specialization. I will now give a brief overview of the major characteristics of these tissue-resident macrophages and their functional roles in pathology and homeostasis. Further consideration of macrophage function has also been done in the later sections of the text when discussing specific diseases and immune responses. Of course the reader should remain aware that a large quantity of our knowledge regarding the roles and function of macrophage is derived from murine studies. While their behavior and characteristics are likely to be broadly similar in humans, there may of course be some subtle, or localized, differences.

2.1.2.1 The Brain

Tissue-resident macrophages within the brain and the central nervous system (CNS) are known as microglia and provide essential functions in maintaining cellular homeostasis and fighting infection. The presence of the blood–brain barrier serves to isolate the CNS from the open passage of substances carried within the bloodstream. This likely includes circulating monocytes and therefore means that most of, and potentially all of, the microglia are derived from prenatal implantation. The presence of the blood–brain barrier also results in the CNS being viewed as an immunologically privileged location.

At the homeostatic level, correct microglial function is crucial for normal brain activity. This is most likely the result of a specific role for microglia in the maintenance of brain synaptic connectivity but may also result from the secretion of neuronal specific growth factors. Activation of the microglia can lead to the induction of inflammation within the brain and the CNS. This is believed to contribute to the development and the pathogenesis of neurodegenerative conditions such as Parkinson's disease and Alzheimer's disease.

2.1.2.2 The Spleen

The functional attributes of the spleen as a filter of the blood and a primer of T- and B-cell responses is made possible predominantly because of the various different macrophage populations that it houses. These macrophage subpopulations are positioned in spatially distinct locations from which they provide specific homeostatic functions. For example, red pulp macrophages recycle iron within the host and are therefore crucial for the phagocytosis and breakdown of unwanted erythrocytes and the retrieval of hemoglobin free in the blood. In contrast, macrophages located in the marginal zone—the boundary between the red and white pulp—are particularly important for the removal of blood-borne pathogens and apoptotic cells. They consequently possess a wide range of cell surface PRRs. Meanwhile, the macrophages in the white pulp itself are principally involved in actually initiating the adaptive response to blood-borne infection.

2.1.2.3 The Bones

We are all familiar with the concept of bone marrow and the importance this plays in hematopoietic functions to maintain the populations of white and red blood cells in the circulation. It is, however, easy to forget that the bones are in fact highly vascularized structures that undergo a continual and dynamic remodeling process to maintain an excellent strength to weight ratio. Key to this constant remodeling are osteoclasts, bone-resident tissue macrophages, which are important for the resorption of bone material. Unbalanced and excessive osteoclast function can contribute to the development of osteoporosis.

2.1.2.4 The Lungs

The lungs, in a manner similar to the intestines, present a unique immunological challenge. The physiological nature of our respiratory system means that the lungs are continually exposed to a wide repertoire of potentially harmful and damaging substances. These include pathogens; particulate material of varying sizes such as dust, diesel fumes, and other products of combustion; and allergens such as animal dander and pollens. The importance of maintaining a healthy environment in the lung is seen through the potentially fatal consequences of diseases and conditions such as pneumonia, acute inflammatory responses such as those induced by asthmatic and allergic episodes, and chronic inflammation as occurs with asbestosis and emphysema. Macrophages in the lung, which are positioned in the alveolae and hence referred to as alveolar macrophages, play a vital role in controlling and regulating this inflammatory response.

Because of the potentially fatal consequences of excessive inflammation in the lungs, and the short timeframe over which this danger can manifest, alveolar macrophages are required to strike a careful balance between tolerance and attack. Inert and/or innocuous inhaled particles need to be either ignored or removed in a noninflammatory manner. In contrast, potentially harmful pathogens need to be rapidly identified and dealt with. The ability of alveolar macrophages to successfully perform these two, almost completely contrasting, roles stems from the range of cell surface receptors they possess and their interactions with epithelial cells in the alveolae. For example, a tolerant noninflammatory phenotype is regulated through interactions with epithelial cells via CD200 and as a result of TGF-β signaling. Similarly, pathogens, allergens, and dying cells can all be recognized and removed in a low-inflammatory, or even noninflammatory, manner through the function of pulmonary surfactant–associated proteins on the macrophage surface. Disruption of the function of these surfactant-associated proteins immediately results in the induction of chronic inflammation.

The key surfactants recognized by the surfactant-associated proteins on the surface of the alveolar macrophages are the collectins and surfactant proteins A and D. These proteins bind carbohydrates on the pathogen surface and prime them for phagocytosis. They are highly similar to the recognition proteins used by the lectin pathway of complement activation (see Section 3.4.3), but fortunately, given the inflammatory capacity of complement, do not have the ability to switch on complement-mediated signaling pathways.

Somewhat surprisingly and possibly counterintuitively the broadly antiinflammatory phenotype of alveolar macrophages is maintained even when they are dealing with the presence of pathogens. They are highly efficient at phagocytosing bacteria, but achieve this without inducing a generalized inflammatory response. In response to viral infection, alveolar macrophages act as an important source of type I interferon, which serves to place neighboring cells into an antiviral state less permissive to subsequent infection. In addition, they provide important functions necessary for the restoration and repair of damaged lung tissues.

2.1.2.5 The Liver

Liver-specific macrophages are known as Kupffer cells. The role of the liver in important metabolic processes and detoxification shows that Kupffer cells are heavily exposed to antigens in the bloodstream. These antigens can originate from a range of different sources, including foods, medicines, and pathogens. Kupffer cells display high levels of phagocytic activity, even for macrophages. They are present at highest concentration in the regions of the liver that first receives the circulating blood. This improves their efficacy at filtering and screening the blood, which is especially important for success in removing circulating pathogens. Indeed, microbial counts in the liver (as well as in the spleen) are often used as a marker of infection burden in animal models of disease.

In addition to providing protection against blood-borne pathogens, Kupffer cells are also important for the clearance of a range of potentially harmful molecules from the circulation. These include the products of dead and dying cells, immune complexes, components of the extracellular matrix, and particles that have been coated in complement or fibronectin. Kupffer cells also help to control the level of lipoproteins in the blood. In particular, they extract low-density lipoproteins (LDLs) from the circulation following the interaction of LDL with LDL receptors on the surface of the Kupffer cell. These LDLs are then broken down in the macrophage by catabolic pathways. In a manner analogous to the macrophages found in the red pulp of the spleen, Kupffer cells have an important role in the recycling of iron in the host. This is achieved through two main routes and is facilitated by the surface expression of particular scavenger receptors on the macrophage plasma membrane. For example, CD163 allows the active capture of hemoglobin-containing complexes, whereas other receptors aid the capture and internalization of damaged or senescent erythrocytes.

2.1.3 Dendritic Cells

The dendritic cell (DC) was first discovered in the 1970s by Ralph Steinman and Zanvil Cohn, for which Steinman shared the 2011 Nobel Prize in Physiology and Medicine. In many ways the DC is the key cell in facilitating the ability of an organism to mount a highly specific adaptive immune response to antigen and I will discuss in more detail the role of DCs in bridging the innate/adaptive interface in Section 5.

DCs are a highly polymorphic and heterogeneous type of cell but can be broadly segregated into two main types—conventional DCs (cDCs) and plasmacytoid DCs (pDCs). pDCs are similar to B-cell–derived plasma cells in appearance and are found both in the blood and lymphoid tissues. A major role of pDCs appears to be in the detection of viral infection upon viral-induced PRR stimulation, especially of TLR7 and TLR9, these cells produce phenomenal levels of the type I interferon IFNα, which serves to induce an antiviral state in surrounding cells and tissues. cDCs encompass all other types of DC and represent those first identified by Steinman. They are found in nonlymphoid as well as lymphoid tissues and are crucial in the induction of immunity to foreign antigens and the maintenance of tolerance against host-derived antigens. These functions result from their exceptional ability to sample their surroundings and specifically phagocytose material, efficient processing and presentation of these antigens to T cells, and ability to activate T cells upon antigen recognition.

2.1.4 Neutrophils

Neutrophils are the most abundant type of leukocyte and, in humans, can constitute in the region of 40–60% of the circulating white blood cell count. The lifespan of a circulating human neutrophil is short and may only be in the region of 8–12 h. However, there is suggestion, albeit yet to be widely validated or accepted, that some human neutrophils can survive for almost five and a half days in the circulation. What is clear is that neutrophils that migrate out of the circulation to a site of infection, damage, or inflammation see an associated increase in their lifespan and routinely survive for a few days. In response to infection, cellular damage, and sterile inflammation, neutrophil numbers in the circulation increase. This is the result of neutrophils being released from the bone marrow, in which they are constitutively created from myeloid precursors, in response to the receipt of chemotactic signals, which include IL-8, leukotriene B4, and the complement anaphylatoxin fragment C5a. The process of neutrophil generation within the bone marrow is under the control of granulocyte colony stimulating factor, which itself is regulated by IL-17A produced from γδ T cells and natural killer (NK) cells. Changes in neutrophil number within the circulation, often measured in terms of the neutrophil to leukocyte ratio, are commonly used as a quick check for the presence of active or recent infection.

The neutrophil itself, like other granulocytes, has a multilobed nucleus and contains a large number of cytoplasmic granules (Fig. 2.1). These cytoplasmic granules can be split into three different types based on their order of production during neutrophil synthesis and also on their contents. These are often referred to as primary, secondary, and tertiary granules but can also be called azurophilic, specific, and gelatinase granules, respectively (Fig. 2.1). The contents of these granules are proinflammatory in nature and play a key role in the ability of neutrophils to kill both internalized and extracellular bacteria. Granule composition has to vary because many of the proteases produced would degrade one another if they were contained within the same location. Primary granules

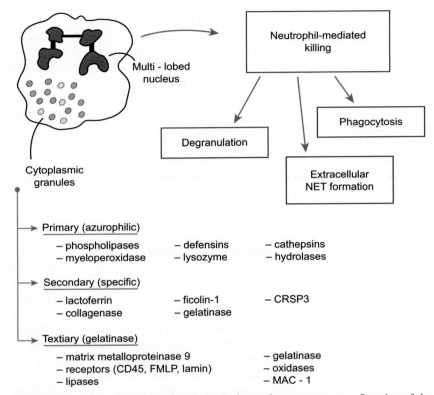

FIGURE 2.1   **Neutrophils and their role in the innate immune response.** Overview of the major morphological features of neutrophils, their mechanisms of killing, and some of the contents of the three major types of cytoplasmic granules they possess.

are peroxide positive and contain myeloperoxidase and in some instances anti-microbial peptides of the defensin family. Secondary granules in contrast are peroxidase negative and instead are split into numerous categories depending on their major constituent. The most common types of secondary granule are those enriched in gelatinase, ficolin-1, lactoferrin, or cysteine-rich secretory protein 3. Tertiary granules contain matrix metalloproteinase 9.

The extremely hostile and inflammatory composition of the cytoplasmic granules in a neutrophil presents a threat not only to internalized or extracellular bacteria but also to the host tissues. Release of granule contents into the extra-cellular space will lead to host tissue damage and therefore needs to be care-fully controlled and limited. An excessive or an unregulated neutrophil response can potentially lead to unwanted damage to host tissues, can delay the onset of the processes of resolution and repair, or alternatively may contribute to chronic inflammation. With such a short lifespan, it is vital that the process of neutrophil death is carefully controlled to stop the unintentional release of these potentially harmful molecules. Consequently, neutrophils are preconditioned to undergo controlled cell death, i.e., apoptosis (see Section 3.5.1), in a constitutive manner. This enables the uncontrolled release of granule contents to be minimized and facilitates the phagocytosis of dying neutrophils by macrophages at the site of inflammation or in the liver or spleen. Delays in the initiation of constitutive apoptosis may contribute to enhanced or poorly controlled inflammation. However, following migration out of the circulation, this process is deliberately slowed down to allow neutrophils time to perform their immune functions.

2.1.4.1 Migration From the Circulation

Neutrophils are commonly the first immune cells recruited to a site of infection or damage and are one of the major effector cells in terms of providing the initial inflammatory response to contain and control the threat. It is therefore important that neutrophils are able to rapidly move from the circulation to the site of infection or damage. This process is known as extravasation—departure from the vascular system.

Extravasation is a multistep process that involves specific interactions between the neutrophil and endothelial cells lining the blood vessels. The general process is followed by most types of leukocytes to enable their migration to specific tissues from the circulation. The key stages are generally referred to as rolling, adhesion, crawling, and transmigration. The elements of each stage in the context of neutrophil extravasation are summarized below:

- *Rolling*: Neutrophils traveling in the circulation need to be captured to enable their recruitment to sites of inflammation in the tissues. This process is started by changes in the surface composition of the vascular endothelium brought about by the action of inflammatory mediators released from the inflamed tissue. These commonly include histamines, leukotrienes, and cytokines and are often derived from tissue-resident leukocytes, such as macrophages, which have detected the presence of either endogenous or exogenous danger signals. The endothelial cells increase their expression of adhesion molecules including P-selectin and E-selectin (Fig. 2.2), which then interact with glycoproteins on the surface of the circulating neutrophils. Similarly, L-selectin on the neutrophil surface interacts with endothelial glycoproteins. This part of the process is known as tethering, anchors the neutrophils to the endothelium, and then allows them to slowly roll along the endothelium surface by continually making and breaking these adhesive contacts.
- *Adhesion*: Full adhesion of the neutrophil occurs in response to a gradient of chemoattractants, such as IL-8, which are deposited on the vascular surface as they migrate from the source of inflammation or infection. The chemoattractants interact with the appropriate G-protein coupled receptor (GPCR) on the surface of the neutrophil and this helps stimulate interactions between the integrins intercellular adhesion molecule 1 (ICAM1) (Fig. 2.2) and vascular cell adhesion molecule 1 (VCAM1) on the endothelium with their cognate-binding partners lymphocyte function-associated antigen 1

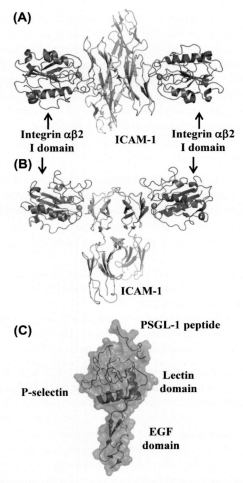

(A)

↑ **Integrin αβ2 I domain** **ICAM-1** ↑ **Integrin αβ2 I domain**

(B) ↓ ↓

ICAM-1

(C) **PSGL-1 peptide**

Lectin domain

P-selectin

EGF domain

FIGURE 2.2 **Example structures of proteins involved in cell adhesion processes.** Top (A) and side (B) views of ICAM-1 (sand and green) in complex with the I domain from integrin αβ2 (blue) (PDB 1MQ8). The magnesium iron observed at the interface between the two proteins is represented as a *pale purple sphere*. (C) Surface and cartoon representations of the structure of P-selectin (blue) bound to a peptide from P-selection glycoprotein ligand 1 (PSGL-1) (red) (PDB 1G1S).

(LFA1) and very late antigen 4 (VLA4) on the neutrophil. These are strong interactions that serve to firmly adhere the neutrophil to the endothelial cell surface.

- *Crawling*: Protein conformational changes lead to alterations in integrin binding and result in a preference for ICAM1 to interact with macrophage-1 antigen (MAC1) on the neutrophil surface. This allows the movement of the neutrophil toward high concentrations of chemoattractants. As mentioned earlier, IL-8 is a major attractant for neutrophils. Other molecules that act as chemoattractants include C5a, C3a, leukotriene B4 and the bacterial product *N*-formylmethionyl-leucyl phenylalanine (fMLP).

- *Transmigration*: This is the actual process of movement either between, or through, endothelial cells by the neutrophil to enable exit from the circulation and entry into the surrounding tissue. The entire process takes between 10 and 20 min, if transit occurs between cells, and between 20 and 30 min, if the neutrophil moves through a cell. Transmigration is heavily reliant on integrins and other cell adhesion molecules and involves cytoskeletal changes in the endothelial cells to permit neutrophil passage. Once in the tissues the neutrophils migrate to the site at which they are needed and this again occurs in response to chemotactic gradients.

2.1.4.2 Neutrophil-Driven Bacterial Killing

Neutrophils can kill bacteria by three main processes: phagocytosis, degranulation, and through the formation of extracellular traps (Fig. 2.1). Pathogens that come into contact with neutrophils are phagocytosed and then killed within the endosomes. This can be mediated either through the action of ROS, or as a result of the fusion of the endosome with cytoplasmic granules and the release and activity of lytic enzymes such as lysozyme, defensins, and cathepsin proteases. Degranulation simply involves the release of granule contents into the extracellular environment where they become free to interact with, damage, and destroy extracellular pathogens. This process may be stimulated by neutrophil–pathogen contact, which helps locate the granule contents proximal to the target, but obviously has the potential for inflicting damage to surrounding host tissue as well. The third method of pathogen killing employed by neutrophils occurs through the production of neutrophil extracellular traps (NETs).

Formation of a NET is a terminal process for the neutrophil as it involves the extracellular release of neutrophil DNA in the form of chromatin filaments. These chromatin filaments, which are approximately 15–17 nm in diameter, provide the organizational scaffold for NET formation. Mitochondrial DNA can also be released and contribute to NET formation. The DNA is covered in proteins, which include histones, proteases, and many components found in the cytoplasmic granules. The release of DNA to create a NET can occur after the receipt of pathogen-associated molecular pattern (PAMP)-mediated signals through PRRs or as part of the process of cell lysis. It involves ROS activation and the degradation of the nuclear envelope. NET structures are able to trap and capture bacteria and other pathogens and given the composition of the proteins coating the DNA strands are likely to result in direct pathogen killing. NETs are also able to act as molecular alarm signals—through the combination of danger/damage-associated molecular pattern (DAMPs) and PAMPs they contain—to activate PRR-mediated immune signaling. They have also been suggested to play a role in the pathogenesis of chronic inflammatory conditions such as atherosclerosis and psoriasis.

2.1.5 Eosinophils

Just like neutrophils, eosinophils are a type of granulocyte. They contribute only a small fraction, usually 1–4%, of leukocytes in the peripheral circulation and are most commonly located in lymphoid organs and mucosal tissues. Their presence in the mucosa is integral to their ability to provide an extremely rapid response to infections, allergens, and other sources of cellular danger.

Eosinophils contain a large number of cytoplasmic granules that are pre-loaded with a wide variety of specific effector molecules enabling them to immediately release the contents of the granules upon activation without the need for either transcriptional or translational upregulation. The mechanism by which granule contents are released (degranulation) depends on both the manner and the degree of activation. Degranulation can occur as a result of the exocytosis of granule contents, programmed and controlled eosinophil cytolysis, or most commonly a process known as piecemeal degranulation. This latter mechanism allows the controlled and specific emptying on certain granules into the extracellular space. The decision as to which granules are emptied and released is determined by the range of activation signals received by the eosinophil. Migration of granules to the plasma membrane is followed by the fusion of the granule and plasma membranes in a process driven by soluble N-ethylmaleimide-sensitive-factor attachment protein receptor (SNARE) proteins. This leads to the extracellular release of a biologically and functionally diverse range of molecules that includes the following:

- Cationic peptides and proteins—These represent the major granule components and include proteins such as major basic proteins, eosinophilic cationic protein, and various RNAses (Fig. 2.3). They are often directly cytolytic either as a result of interaction with cell-surface receptors or through direct destabilization of the target pathogens membrane. For example, major basic proteins contain a high proportion of basic amino acids such as arginine and lysine. This allows direct interaction with negatively charged membranes and subsequently destabilizes membrane integrity leading to permeabilization and/or destruction of target cells.
- Cytokines and chemokines—Eosinophils are often associated with type 2 immune responses and therefore unsurprisingly possess granules containing classical type 2 mediators such as IL-4, IL-5, and IL-13. However, they also secrete type 1–associated cytokines such as IL-2, IL-12, IFNγ, and TGFβ. The eosinophils themselves express surface receptors responsive to both classifications of cytokine thereby highlighting their functional diversity.
- Lipid mediators—A variety of immunologically competent lipids have been identified in eosinophil granules. These include leukotrienes and eicosanoids, some of which have been directly associated with eosinophil-associated exacerbation of asthma.
- Growth factors—The secretion of harmful cytolytic molecules contributes to immune defense, but also has the potential to contribute to immunopathology

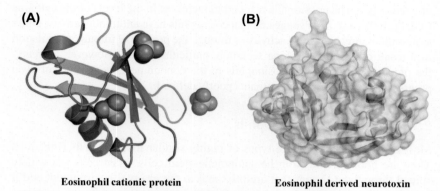

Eosinophil cationic protein   **Eosinophil derived neurotoxin**

FIGURE 2.3   **Structures of eosinophil granule contents.** Structure of the (A) eosinophil cationic protein and (B) eosinophil-derived neurotoxin, also known as RNAse3. The position of sulfate
ions are shown as *spheres* in panel (A) and may represent the potential binding site for proteoglycan
molecules.

by causing significant levels of harm to surrounding tissues and cells. Through
the release of growth factors such as platelet-derived growth factor (PDGF) and
vascular endothelial growth factor (VEGF), eosinophils are able to contribute to
the process of tissue remodeling and the restoration of homeostasis.

Eosinophil function is associated with allergic and antihelminth immune
processes. Granule secretions and eosinophils are commonly found at sites of
allergic responses in the bronchial and intestinal mucosal surfaces. This occurs,
for example, during atopic asthma or eosinophilic gastroenteritis. Eosinophils
are also present in the skin lesions associated with conditions such as atopic dermatitis. In all of these conditions the eosinophils are widely believed to contribute to both pathological and repair processes. Eosinophil-mediated targeting of
helminths can result in direct parasite death via the action of cytolytic peptides,
or through combined action with complement and antibody-based defenses. In
addition, the secretion of cytokines such as IL-4 helps to drive the localized
immune environment toward a type 2 antihelminth response.

In addition to their well-defined roles in allergy and helminth-targeted
responses, it has become clear that eosinophils also have important contributions
to make in the innate response to bacterial and viral infection, and even against
tumor cells. Bacteria are efficient activators of eosinophils and are directly targeted for eosinophil-mediated killing. This can be through the action of cationic
peptides, or via extracellular deposits, which are formed from secretions of protein and mitochondrial DNA from the eosinophils. These deposits then trap and
immobilize the bacteria, thereby aiding their killing and removal by other immune
mediators. Eosinophil-derived RNAses contribute to their antiviral functionality.
This is further helped by the presence of PRRs, such as TLR7, which respond to
viral ssRNA ligands. Direct recruitment of eosinophils to tumors occurs as a result

of chemotaxis. The eosinophils respond to increases in the levels of the cytokine CCL11. It has also been suggested that eosinophils have antitumor activity, either as a result of direct cytolytic activity or through the process of immunomodulation as a result of specific cytokine secretion, particularly IL-4. However, currently the precise contribution of eosinophils to the containment, regression, or even progression, of tumor growth remains poorly defined.

2.1.6 Mast Cells and Basophils

Mast cells and basophils are types of highly similar myeloid cells (Fig. 2.1). They are both derived from hematopoietic stem cells. Mast cells are widely spread throughout tissues that are proximal to the external environment and it is in these locations that they undergo final maturation. Basophils are much less common. They mature in the bone marrow and migrate to tissues when needed in response to the presence of chemical mediators such as IL-3 and thymic stromal lymphopoietin. Basophils are short lived, normally surviving for between 1 and 3 days. Mast cells in contrast are long lived as they have the capability to undergo further proliferation in response to appropriate mitogenic stimuli. Both mast cells and basophils have high surface levels of the high-affinity IgE receptor FcεRI. Coupled with their surface proximal location, this makes mast cells in particular one of the first immune cells to come into contact with pathogens, toxins, and antigens. This helps explain their important contributions in the innate immune response to, for example, allergens and venoms.

Mast cells and basophils are often key components in the rapid response of individuals to allergens and may indeed have an important role in the progression of anaphylactic shock. Activation of mast cells and basophils can be either antigen or antibody (IgE) dependent. Activation occurs when a few of the high-affinity FcεRI receptors become aggregated following antigen recognition by IgE prebound to the FcεRI receptors. The high affinity of the FcεRI receptor means that individual mast cells and basophils can be activated by a variety of different allergenic stimuli simultaneously. This results in a complex process of cellular degranulation and the release of inflammatory mediators such as histamine, heparin, proteoglycans, proteases, and cytokines. This process is extremely quick and can occur just minutes after the initial exposure. The degree of mediator secretion is related to the strength of the activating stimulus, meaning that high allergenic loads produce more extensive degranulation and consequently are potentially more dangerous to the individual.

Mast cells also contribute to the host response to infection. As a general rule, mast cell activation enhances the protective elements of the host immune response to parasites, bacteria, and viruses. Parasites can activate mast cells through antigen- or antibody-dependent pathways in a manner similar to allergens. This can aid direct parasite killing through the action of secreted tryptase, as well as stimulate the expulsion of intestinal parasites via IL-4 and IL-13–mediated pathways. Bacteria and viruses do not generally result in antibody-dependent activation of mast cells, but instead, these pathogens activate mast cells through the stimulation of PRRs, the work of complement, or recognition of endogenous markers of endothelial stress and cellular damage such as endothelin 1. Mast cell activation by these routes does not generally induce rapid wholesale degranulation but rather a more controlled and limited secretion of molecules. These molecules can include CCL2, CCL4, and CXCL8 that act as chemoattractants for other immune cells, such as neutrophils. Activated mast cells also show an increase in their phagocytic function. Overall, the balance between mast cell–induced immunopathology and protection is a fine one and in many cases is intrinsically linked to the quantity of activatory stimulus and hence the level of mast cell activation that occurs.

2.1.7 Innate Lymphoid Cells

Classically, lymphocytes are the cornerstone of adaptive immunity and were historically viewed as being entirely separate from the workings of the innate immune response. The identification of NK cells in 1975 provided the first evidence that lymphocytes also had an important role to play in the innate response to infection. In the subsequent years, extensive research has highlighted the essential need for APCs to be primed by innate immune activation in order to efficiently induce protective adaptive immunity. It is now clear that the innate immune response plays an integral and essential function in driving the development and progression of the adaptive response—the two systems are integrally linked (see Section 5). In addition, knowledge of the range and diversity of lymphocytes involved in the innate immune response has blossomed. This has resulted in the identification of lymphocytes that function in innate immunity. Phenotypically these innate lymphoid cells (ILCs) provide functional cellular parallels for the major proportion of the adaptive T-cell phenotypes. This similarity is not necessarily surprising given that both innate and adaptive lymphocytes are ultimately derived from the same population of precursor cells—the common lymphoid progenitor. The precise microenvironment of the progenitor cells dictates the lineage they commit to. Notch ligands and bone morphogenic proteins play an important role in driving them toward an innate phenotype. Once a commitment has been made to the innate pathway, these cells will then develop into either NK progenitors and subsequently NK cells or into common helper innate lymphoid progenitors, from which they will develop into one of the three types of ILC. The final maturation steps are influenced by microbial and dietary factors including retinoic acid, a metabolite of vitamin D produced by a range of cell types and compounds that activate the aryl hydrocarbon receptor.

NK cells can be described as the innate equivalent of cytotoxic T cells, while the same is true for ILC1, ILC2, and ILC3 cells and their respective adaptive T cell Th1, Th2, and Th17 counterparts. The increasing number of innate lymphocyte types has led to their proposed classification into three discrete types

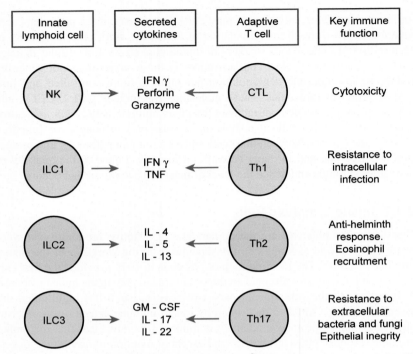

FIGURE 2.4 **Innate lymphoid cells (ILCs).** Schematic diagram showing the relationship between ILCs and T cells, the principle cytokines they secrete, and their main effector functionality.

based on their function, pattern of differentiation, the transcription factors they express, and the effector cytokines they secrete (Fig. 2.4). However, as our understanding and knowledge of ILCs is still somewhat in its infancy, there is currently much debate as to how to best describe these cells and their functional relationships with the adaptive T-cell phenotypes. There is therefore a high probability that the current classifications may well change in the future. The major characteristics of ILCs are described below.

2.1.7.1 Natural Killer Cells

NK cells were first thought to be a form of granulocyte because of the presence of cytoplasmic granules. However, they are in fact a type of innate lymphocyte and are highly important in the innate defense against pathogens and tumors. To operate effectively, NK cells require activation by exposure to cytokines such as IL-2, -12, -15, -18, and IFNγ.

At the simplest level the activation of NK cells works on a basis of "missing-self." MHC class I acts as an inhibitory receptor on NK cells and serves to inactivate their killing responses against a target cell. Consequently, cells that do not express MHC class I, as often occurs in tumor cells and as a result of viral infection, are unable to stop NK activation upon engagement and therefore become a target for killing. However, the system is actually somewhat more complex and involves a variety of activating receptors and signals—which stimulate NK-cell–mediated killing—working in conjunction with inhibitory receptors and signals—whose role is to stop NK cell activation. Examples of activating receptors include the NK cell lectin-like receptor NKG2D, which responds to endogenous surface markers such as MICA (MHC class I polypeptide-related sequence A) and UL16 binding proteins (ULBP) 1-6 that are upregulated in response to cellular stress; the FcγR receptor that stimulates antibody-dependent cell cytotoxicity; and the SLAM (signaling lymphocytic activation molecule) family of receptors that tend to interact with themselves on the surface of the target cell. The majority of the NK cell inhibitory receptors work by binding to MHC class I. In humans this function is provided by a family of killer cell immunoglobulin-like receptors (KIRs), whereas mice use the Ly49 family. These inhibitory receptors display different levels of affinity for the polymorphic MHC I molecule. Inhibition of NK cell activation by KIR or Ly49 engagement involves phosphorylation of intracellular tyrosine residues in the receptor cytoplasmic regions and the recruitment of specific phosphatases, which inhibit activatory signaling pathways.

When an NK cell is activated, it often mediates cell death through the induction of apoptotic pathways in the target cell. This can occur in a number of ways. The NK cell produces molecules such as TRAIL (TNF-related apoptosis-inducing ligand) and CD95-L, which then engage death receptors on the surface of the target cell and trigger the extrinsic pathway of apoptosis (see Section 3.5). An activated NK cell also secretes a wide range of cytolytic enzymes that target and permeabilize the membrane of the target cell. This disrupts homeostatic balance and allows molecules into the cell, both of which can serve as further triggers of apoptosis. The induction of apoptotic death is important to limit the degree of inflammation. Activated NK cells serve as an important source of the proinflammatory cytokine IFNγ, which is especially important for stimulating macrophage effector functions. There is an increasing amount of evidence that some NK cells, although inherently an innate effector cell, are able to persist and develop some form of memory capability thereby placing them directly in the interface between the innate and adaptive responses.

2.1.7.2 Type I Innate Lymphoid Cells

Type I ILCs have many similarities with NK cells. They are also activated by the action of the cytokines IL-12, -15, and -18, in response to intracellular infections and tumor cells. Just as is the case for NK cells, this also causes them to secrete IFNγ, but unlike NK cells, they are not directly cytotoxic and instead, also secrete TNFα. This has the net result of stimulating macrophage activation and the production of oxygen radicals, both of which are important defenses against intracellular infection. ILC1 cells drive a type 1 immune response and help promote the development and maturation of the adaptive response. They are thought to potentially contribute to the pathology of a number of forms of inflammatory bowel disease.

2.1.7.3 Type II Innate Lymphoid Cells

Type II ILCs are activated by cytokines that are produced by damaged epithelial cells. These are commonly released in response to the presence of helminths, by the action of allergens or as a result of tissue injury. The cytokines secreted by activated ILC2 cells are classic type 2 cytokines (Fig. 2.4). They stimulate the process of vasodilation, the production of mucus, and repair to damaged tissues and the extracellular matrix and can influence the host's thermal regulation. ILC2 cells still activate macrophages, but the pathway differs from that used by ILC1 cells. ILC2 cells provide protection against fat-induced inflammatory responses and may also protect against the development of metabolic syndromes, insulin resistance, and diabetes. An inability to produce ILC2 cells leads to increased pathogenicity upon infection with the parasites *Nippostrongylus brasiliensis* and *Schistosoma mansoni*.

2.1.7.4 Type III Innate Lymphoid Cells

Type III ILCs become activated as a result of exposure to IL-1β and IL-23 produced in response to infection. This in turn causes the ILC3 cells to secrete IL-17, IL-22, and GM-CSF themselves. This stimulates phagocytic processes, the secretion of antimicrobial peptides, and improved epithelial cell survival. Intestinal ILC3 cells are reliant on the host microbiota to develop properly. Pathologically, ILC3 cells are important contributors to fat-induced inflammation and therefore can be considered as working in a manner opposite to ILC2 cells in this context. ILC3 cells have also been connected with the immunopathology of inflammatory bowel disease and colitis.

All ILCs respond quickly to infection or injury. Their influence in directing the final direction of the immune response along particular pathways makes them an attractive target for immunomodulation. Disruption or alteration of ILC function could be used to alter or modify the immune response that arises in response to chronic inflammation, vaccination, or as a general means of controlling the immune response.

2.1.8 Gamma-Delta (γδ) T Cells

T lymphocytes can be defined by the combination of T-cell receptor (TCR) chains that they express on their surface. The majority of T cells express α and β chains and are therefore classed as αβ T cells but normally referred to as just T cells. However, some T cells express a TCR composed of γ and δ chains. These cells are consequently known as γδ T cells and they represent a subset of T lymphocytes that possess attributes bridging the innate/adaptive divide. The functionality of classical αβ T cells only becomes apparent following stimulation and clonal expansion. However, γδ T cells are found in the peripheral tissues, not just the primary lymphoid organs, and are able to mediate various effector functions within a matter of hours, i.e., over the timescale of an innate response. Their functional characteristics can be broadly broken down into six areas, which include the following:

- Production of granzymes to bring about the direct lysis of damaged, stressed, or infected cells.
- Modulation of immune cell function by the secretion of a wide range of cytokines and chemokines, such as IFNγ to influence local immune effects and IL-13 to drive systemic immunity.
- The facilitation of IgE production from B cells.
- Presentation of antigens to prime αβ T cells for the adaptive response.
- Stimulation of DC maturation.
- Production of growth factors aimed at controlling the function of stromal cells.

The importance of γδ T cells in the innate immune response has been clearly demonstrated using mice that lack the *Tcrd* gene, which encodes for the T cell δ chain. Consequently, these mice are unable to produce γδ T cells. When exposed to a range of bacterial, viral, and parasitic pathogens including the global killers tuberculosis (*Mycobacterium* spp.) and malaria (*Plasmodium* spp.), these mice become more vulnerable to infection. There appears not to be one specific reason why mice lacking γδ T cells are more susceptible to infection and a variety of immune defects have been observed. These include defects in IFNγ production, failure to prime cytotoxic T cells, and a lack of rapid and early IL-17 secretion. The diverse functionality of γδ T cells positions them uniquely in the immune repertoire and without question, their importance in driving and balancing the immune response will be clearer as research into their function expands further.

2.2 PATTERN RECOGNITION RECEPTOR SIGNALING PATHWAYS

The recognition of conserved molecular structures and patterns is relevant throughout the immune system and underpins a significant proportion of the functionality of the innate immune response. Surface-bound and internal protein receptors whose role it is to recognize and respond to specific molecular structures and patterns are widely distributed across host cells and tissues. These PRRs can be found in many different cell types and show cell-specific patterns of expression but are most commonly expressed on immune cells. The precise pattern and level of receptor expression varies depending on where the cells are located, the likelihood of them coming into contact with potential ligands, the nature of the ligands encountered, and the physiological role of the cell. Macrophages, for example, express a wide range of PRRs, both internally and on their surface, reflecting their importance in the detection of danger and the initiation of protective innate immune defenses.

2.2.1 Pattern Recognition Receptors Recognize Exogenous and Endogenous Dangers

The host is under continual bombardment from potential dangers. Physical and chemical barriers (see Section 1.3.1) provide an excellent and highly effective mechanism by which exogenous dangers are deflected, diverted, and neutralized. They are, however, not perfect and can be breached in many ways such as through the result of barrier dysfunction, traumatic injury, excessive exposure to exogenous dangers, or through injections, surgery, and other deliberate actions. All of this results in the subsequent need for these dangers to be rapidly recognized by the host to facilitate initiation of the correct, most efficient, and appropriate immune defense to neutralize, limit, or remove the threat. We tend to think of exogenous dangers as consisting of bacteria, viruses, fungi, and parasites. Indeed, these pathogenic microorganisms are a major immune threat and contribute extensively to human morbidity and mortality. For example, the World Health Organization reports that both HIV and diarrheal diseases caused 1.5 million deaths each, worldwide in 2012. However, the innate immune system also has to deal with nonpathogenic exogenous dangers. These include allergens, toxins, poisons, venoms, and particulate materials such as diesel fumes, asbestos, and silica particles, which when internalized in the lung can cause extensive chronic inflammation, damage, and even death.

Many researchers originally held the view that the role of PRRs was to detect, and initiate a response to, exogenous pathogens, i.e., contribute to the discrimination of self versus nonself. While this remains an important, and may be the primary role, of PRRs, it is by no means their only role. In Section 1.1.2 the "danger" theory of innate immunity was also introduced, and we saw that in essence the function of the (innate) immune system is to identify both actual and potential cellular damage. This then results in the initiation of signaling pathways that will result in removal of the threat, resolution of damage, and restoration of cellular homeostasis. Consequently, as researchers have driven forward our understanding of how PRRs are activated, it has become apparent that a wide range of endogenously derived cellular components can function as "danger" or "damage" signals and are therefore recognized by, and activate, PRRs. Examples of endogenously derived activators of the innate immune response include high concentrations of extracellular ATP, cellular efflux of potassium, damaged mitochondria, uric acid, cholesterol crystals, heat-shock proteins, and high-mobility box group proteins.

The PRRs that recognize both exogenous and endogenous PAMPs and DAMPs can be broadly split into those that are membrane bound (either internally or at the plasma membrane) and those that are cytoplasmic. Soluble PRRs also exist but will not be discussed here because of limitations of space. PRRs display a surprising level of functional redundancy thereby ensuring that threats to the host are not readily missed. The signaling pathways activated by different PRRs are often fairly similar at the effector level and commonly centered around the activation of stress kinases, NFκB-regulated genes, interferon-response genes, and inflammatory caspases. There is, however, extensive cross talk between different PRR signaling networks, which enables an exquisite level of danger-specific response to be achieved in many cases. One should image that the contribution of PRR signaling to the innate immune response functions not as a digital system, but as a high-level mixing deck in which hundreds of different signals contribute to differing degrees to the precise cellular response produced.

2.2.2 Domain Organization of the Pattern Recognition Receptors

The global repertoire of PRRs is broad and expansive and they recognize a wide range of different activators. This diversity makes it impossible to define a conserved structural organization observed by all PRRs; however, there are a number of broad organizational similarities between different families of PRR (Fig. 2.5). At the simplest level a PRR requires a domain to detect the appropriate activating stimulus or molecular pattern and an effector domain

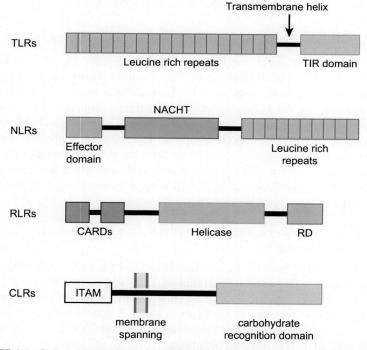

FIGURE 2.5 Pattern recognition receptor domain organization. A simplified schematic of the domain organization of the Toll-like receptor (TLR), nucleotide-binding, leucine-rich repeat–containing receptor (NLR), RIG-I like receptor (RLR), and C-type lectin receptor (CLR) families of pattern recognition receptor. The position of the transmembrane helix and the membrane spanning region of the TLRs and CLRs is marked. The effector domain of the NLRs usually takes the form of either a pyrin domain, a caspase recruitment domain (CARD), or a baculovirus inhibitor repeats domain. The recognition domain (RD) of the RLRs is also sometimes known as a C-terminal domain and is involved in dsRNA recognition, especially of 5'-phosphorylated dsRNA. The CLRs can contain different cytoplasmic domains to the ITAM and multiple carbohydrate recognition domains, or even some form of extracellular ligand-binding domain.

that mediates the protein:protein interactions required for propagation of signal transduction. This organizational structure is observed in a number of major PRR families, including the Toll-like receptors (TLRs), C-type lectin receptors (CLRs), and PYHIN family members. Other PRRs, particularly some of the cytoplasmic PRRs, contain extra domains that often perform important additional functional roles. For example, the nucleotide-binding domain of the nucleotide-binding, leucine-rich repeat–containing receptors (NLRs) is critical in the regulation of receptor activity and also contributes to the formation of large macromolecular signaling complexes.

The sections that follow provide a basic overview of the major PRR signaling pathways. For a number of these receptors a much more expansive description of the mechanisms by which they are activated, how they propagate signaling, and how they mediate innate immune effector mechanisms is provided in later sections, and this is cross-referenced at the appropriate points.

2.2.3 Toll-Like Receptor Signaling

Being the first true membrane-bound PRRs to be discovered, the TLR family has been the subject of an immense amount of scientific research. They are particularly important in the response to both extracellular and endocytosed pathogens and dangers. All TLRs consist of an N-terminal sequence of leucine-rich repeat (LRRs), which are used to recognize and bind to their ligand and interact with one another to form dimeric complexes that propagate signaling. A single alpha helix is used to span the membrane allowing the positioning of the Toll/interleukin-1 resistance (TIR) domain in the cytoplasm, where it can serve as a platform for the recruitment of additional adaptor molecules and the activation of proinflammatory cytokine signaling.

2.2.3.1 Toll-Like Receptors at the Plasma and Endosomal Membrane

TLRs are found in both the plasma membrane and the endosomal membrane. They are most highly expressed on immune cells and tissues that are likely to come into contact with danger signals. However, the pattern of expression varies with cell type and location. For example TLR7, 8, and 9 are highly expressed in pDCs, and although intestinal epithelial cells do express TLR5 this generally occurs only on their basolateral membrane.

There are 10 functional TLRs in humans. TLRs 1, 2, 4, 5, 6, and 10 are all located in the plasma membrane, whereas TLR3, 7, 8, and 9 are endosomal in location. All TLRs appear to signal as at least a dimer, if not even a higher order aggregate. The evidence that dimers are preformed has been provided for TLR9 and this may be the case for most TLRs. However, preformed dimers need to undergo conformational change—this is the result of ligand binding and for some endosomal TLRs involves protein cleavage events—in order to be activated. With the exception of TLR2, which forms heterodimers with either

TLR1 or TLR6, the other TLRs signal as homodimers. TLR4 may also form a complex with CD36, a key receptor in the binding of oxidized LDL (oxLDL).

The TLRs recognize a variety of ligands (Table 2.1). These are predominantly, but not exclusively, of bacterial origin for the receptors located in the plasma membrane, although TLR4 has also been reported to respond to proteins from viral, allergen, and endogenous sources (Table 2.1). The endosomal TLRs on the other hand recognize nucleic acids, often of viral origin. The recognition of ligand and the mechanism of receptor activation for TLR2, TLR4, and TLR5 are described in more detail in Section 4.

TLR3 is activated by dsRNA, and TLR8 responds to degradation products of ssRNA, such as uridine and short ssRNA oligonucleotides (Fig. 2.6), as well as to small chemicals of the imidazoquinoline family. The LRRs of TLR3, consistent with its endosomal location, only bind to their dsRNA ligand at a pH below 6.5. The dsRNA interacts with regions near both the N- and C-terminal LRRs and does not disrupt the TLR3 LRR structure when compared with the unbound LRRs. This interaction does, however, serve to bring together two TLR3 molecules in a classical "m-shaped" structure (Fig. 2.6). This structure positions the cytoplasmic TIRs to facilitate downstream signaling. The LRRs of TLR8

TABLE 2.1 The Major Activating Ligands of Human TLRs

Plasma Membrane Toll-Like Receptors (TLRs)	Activating Ligands
TLR2:TLR1	Triacylated lipopeptides, peptidoglycan (possibly), Pam_3CSK_4
TLR2:TLR6	Diacylated lipopeptides, Pam_2CSK_4
TLR4	Bacterial lipopolysaccharide, heat shock proteins, high-mobility group proteins, fibronectin, Fel d1, proteoglycans
TLR5	Bacterial flagellin (FliC)
TLR10	Component of *Listeria monocytogenes*
Endosomal TLRs	
TLR3	Double-stranded RNA, small RNAs, poly(I:C)
TLR7	Single-stranded RNA, imidazoquinolines, nucleoside analogues
TLR8	Single-stranded RNA, imidazoquinolines, nucleoside analogues
TLR9	Unmethylated CpG rich DNA (common in bacteria and viruses)

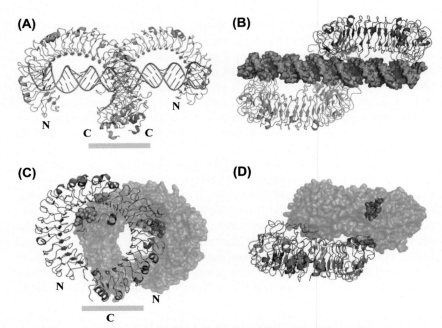

FIGURE 2.6 **The structures of the ligand-bound TLR3 and TLR8 ectodomains.** The ectodomains of two TLR3 proteins form an "m shape" as a result of binding their ligand dsRNA. The
dsRNA makes contacts with both the N-terminal and C-terminal ends of the TLR3 ectodomain and
serves to act as a bridge between the molecules. Both TLR3 molecules have been shown as cartoon
representations with the dsRNA displayed as a cartoon in the side view (A) and a surface representation in the top view (B). (C) Side view and (D) top view of the dimeric complex formed by the TLR8
ectodomains following binding to the breakdown products of ssRNA. Unlike TLR3, dimerization
is mediated by TLR8:TLR8 interactions, which are assisted by the position of the bound uridine
nucleotide (*green spheres*). This is in the same location where synthetic TLR8 ligands from the
imidazoquinoline family bind. The *orange spheres*, which do not contribute to receptor dimerization interfaces, represent the degradation dinucleotide uridine-guanine. Some complexes contained
the RNA sequence UUG at this site. In both side views (A and C) the N and C termini of the ectodomain are labeled, and the approximate position of the membrane is shown by the presence of a *light
blue line*. TLR3 images were generated from PDB 3CIY and the TLR8 images from PDB 4R09.

are cleaved at a point known as the Z-loop between LRRs 14 and 15. However,
the two cleavage products remain associated with one another and consequently
TLR8 also forms an "m-shaped" structure, albeit a more compact one than for
TLR3, in the presence of bound ligand (Fig. 2.6).

2.2.3.2 Toll-Like Receptor Signaling Pathways

Following ligand recognition the induction of a TLR-driven proinflammatory
response requires the formation of a multiprotein signaling complex in the cell
cytoplasm. The first step toward this is the interaction of the TLR TIR dimer
with one of the four immediate downstream adaptor proteins that function in the

TLR signaling cascade. These are myeloid differentiation factor 88 (MyD88), MyD88-adaptor like (Mal), TIR domain–containing adaptor inducing interferon β (TRIF), and TRIF-related adaptor molecule (TRAM). A fifth adaptor, sterile alpha- and armadillo-motif–containing protein, also exists but is a negative regulator of TLR signaling via both TRIF-dependent and MyD88-dependent pathways. In general the TLRs signal via a pathway dependent on MyD88 to activate NFκB-mediated signaling, stress kinase pathways, and/or the expression of type I interferons. This can be mediated via direct interaction between the TIR domains of the TLR and of MyD88, as occurs with TLR5, for example. It can also first involve recruitment of the bridging adaptor Mal, which then recruits MyD88. This approach is used by TLR4 and, under certain circumstances, has been reported for TLR2, 7, 8, and 9. TLR4 can also recruit TRAM to its TIR, which in turn brings in TRIF and leads the induction of a type I interferon response. TLR3 directly recruits TRIF and then upregulates the transcription factor IRF3 to stimulate the production of the type I interferons IFNα and IFNβ. The signal transduction pathways activated by these pathways have been briefly summarized in Figs. 2.7, 2.8, and 2.9.

2.2.3.2.1 The Myddosome Complex

The key cytoplasmic multiprotein macromolecular complex formed in TLR signaling is known as the Myddosome (Fig. 2.10). This complex connects the activated TLR to the downstream signaling molecules. Myddosome formation requires extensive protein:protein interactions. Key to this are interactions formed between protein folds of the death domain (DD) superfamily—interactions that are found throughout immune and cell death signaling cascades.

The DD superfamily consists of four different, but closely related, helical bundle folds namely the DD, the death effector domain (DED), the pyrin domain (PYD), and the caspase recruitment domain (CARD). Members of the DD family form homotypic interactions, i.e., DD with DD, PYD with PYD, and CARD with CARD, which are based on the presence of three different types of interface on the proteins. These interfaces are known as type I, II, and III and each consists of portions a and b. The interfaces are formed through the interaction between specific but distinct regions of the protein (Fig. 2.10). Consequently, each DD family member has the potential to bind to six other family members. This obviously provides scope to create large multiprotein complexes with variable stoichiometry. For example, in addition to the Myddosome, these interactions drive the formation of the filaments associated with inflammasome activation (see Section 4.2), and various cell death–associated complexes such as the Piddosome, the apoptosome, and the death-inducing signaling complex. Heterotypic interactions between DD family members, which include the DED of pro-caspase-8 and the PYD of ASC and the DD of p75 with the CARD of RIPK2, have been reported.

Formation of the Myddosome begins with the recruitment of MyD88 to the TIR dimer of the activated TLR. This is driven by TIR:TIR interactions and leaves the DD of MyD88 available for further intermolecular interactions with

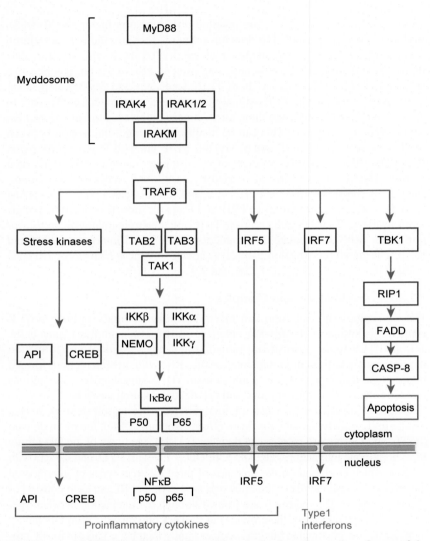

FIGURE 2.7   MyD88-dependent signaling pathways. A schematic overview of some of the major downstream signaling components relevant to the TLR pathway following recruitment of MyD88, its interaction with members of the IRAK family, and the subsequent formation of a Myddosome complex. Interaction of the Myddosome with TRAF6 facilitates multiple different signaling pathways. These include the stress kinase pathways leading to upregulation of the transcription factors AP1 and CREB; activation of the classical NFκB pathway and nuclear translocation of p50 and p65; initiation of caspase-8–dependent apoptosis via RIP1; and activation of the transcription factors IRF5 and IRF7. With the exception of IRF7, which stimulates type I interferons, the other activated transcription factors lead to the production of proinflammatory cytokines.

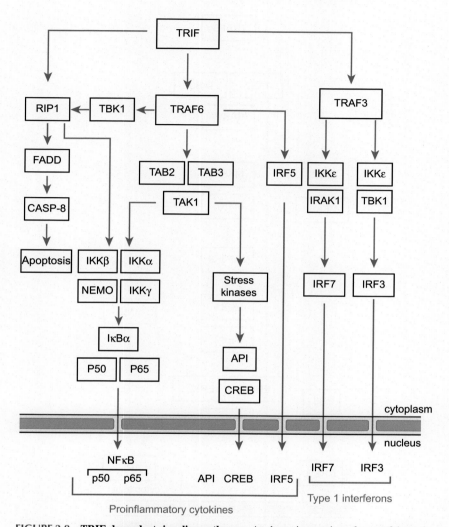

FIGURE 2.8   **TRIF-dependent signaling pathways.** A schematic overview of some of the major downstream signaling components relevant to the TLR pathway following recruitment of the adaptor protein TRIF and hence relevant to TLR3 and TLR4 signaling. There is overlap with some of the signaling cascades of MyD88-dependent TLR signaling, which, given the central involvement of TRAF6 in both pathways, is unsurprising. As with MyD88-dependent signaling, we see activation of the stress kinase pathways leading to upregulation of the transcription factors AP1 and CREB; activation of the classical NFκB pathway and nuclear translocation of p50 and p65; initiation of caspase-8–dependent apoptosis via RIP1; and activation of the transcription factors IRF5 and IRF7. However, there is also upregulation of IRF3, which along with IRF7 stimulates type I interferons. The other activated transcription factors lead to the production of proinflammatory cytokines.

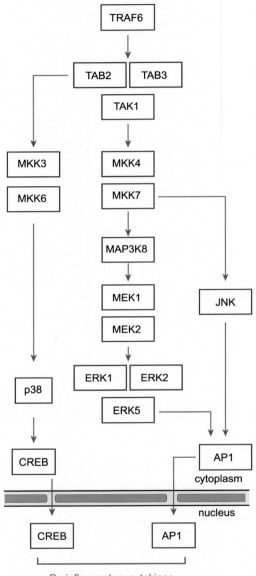

FIGURE 2.9 The stress kinase signaling pathways. Following the activation of the TAB2, TAB3, and TAK1, complex signaling can either lead to canonical NFκB activation or upregulation of the stress kinase pathway. The precise proteins involved in stress kinase signaling varies depending on cell type, nature of the stimuli, and cross talk with other signaling pathways. The transcription factor CREB is activated via an MKK and p38 route, whereas AP1 is activated either via JNK, or via MAPKs and ERKs. The end result is proinflammatory cytokine production.

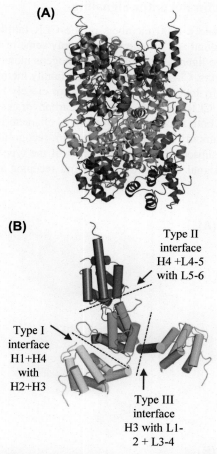

FIGURE 2.10 **The Myddosome.** (A) Crystal structure of the Myddosome signaling complex formed from the death domains of MyD88 (deep red), IRAK4 (green), and IRAK2 (blue). The stoichiometry is 6:4:4. (B) Close-up of the three types of death domain interface as exemplified by the contacts between the death domains of IRAK4 (green) and IRAK4 (yellow)–type I interface; MyD88 (deep red) and IRAK4 (green)—type II interface; and IRAK4 (green) and IRAK4 (cyan)—type III interface. The features of the interface are listed with H=helix and L=loop. The images are generated from PDB 3MOP.

the DDs of members of the IRAK family of protein kinases. The initial interaction appears to occur between MyD88 and IRAK4 followed by the subsequent recruitment of other members of the IRAK family such as IRAK2. The stoichiometry of the complexes that forms appears to be variable, at least in vitro, as purified Myddosomes have been reported with between six and eight MyD88 DDs to four IRAK4 DDs. The situation in vivo is currently unknown. The importance of the Myddosome for TLR signaling is clearly demonstrated by the fact that disruption of the interactions between MyD88 and IRAK4, or between different IRAKS, interferes with and can inhibit TLR signaling.

2.2.4 C-Type Lectin Receptor Signaling

There are approximately 1000 members of the CLR family. This includes a mix of membrane-bound and soluble proteins, only some of which act as PRRs where they recognize ligands from multiple pathogens including fungi, viruses, bacteria, and helminths. Classification as a CLR family member is based on the presence of a carbohydrate recognition domain or closely related protein fold (Fig. 2.11). Not all CLRs actively recognize carbohydrates and the family is split on the basis of both structural and functional characteristics. In relation to the CLRs most commonly associated with pattern-recognition functions, classification into four subsets is done on the basis of the type of signaling motif used to propagate signal transduction following receptor activation. The key

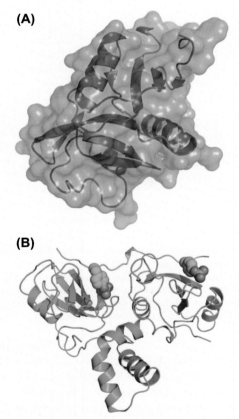

(A)

(B)

FIGURE 2.11 **Structural domains involved in C-type lectin signaling.** (A) The carbohydrate recognition domain of the C-type lectin DC-SIGN. (B) The interaction between the SH2 domains of the intracellular signaling molecule Syk (green) and an ITAM domain (cyan) in which the two critical tyrosine residues have been phosphorylated (*spheres*).

motif is the immunoreceptor tyrosine-based activation motif (ITAM), a short peptide sequence of the form $Yxx(L/I)x_{6-12}Yxx(L/I)$, where x denotes any type of amino acid. The four subsets are known as ITAM, hemITAM, ITAM-coupled, and ITIM receptors. Phosphorylation of the tyrosine (Y) residues plays a key role in signal transduction, as does the recruitment of the kinase Syk. Syk binds directly to canonical ITAMs, but to interact with hemITAMs, two receptors must come together, form a dimer, and create a suitable cytoplasmic scaffold for Syk binding. The actual interaction between the phosphorylated tyrosines and Syk is driven by the two Src homology 2 domains of Syk (Fig. 2.11). Following Syk recruitment the resultant signaling cascades can lead to activation of MAPK, nuclear factor of activated T cells, NFκB, and CARD9.

2.2.4.1 Dectin-1

Dectin-1 belongs to the hemITAM family and can be found in the plasma membrane of various myeloid cells, including DCs, monocytes, and macrophages, as well as B cells. Activation of dectin-1 by fungal cell wall β-glucans stimulates phagocytosis, the production of ROS, and NFκB-mediated cytokine secretion. In contrast to the TLR pathways, dectin-1–mediated NFκB signaling is driven by Syk recruitment and the subsequent formation of a multiprotein signaling complex, the CARD9 signalosome. This signalosome is a tripartite protein complex formed from CARD9, Bcl-10, and MALT-1 and leads to NFκB signaling following activation of p65 and c-Rel.

Dectin-1 activation can also stimulate the cytotoxic responses of neutrophils, improve the efficiency of specific TLR signaling pathways, such as TLR2, and activates the NLRP3 inflammasome following pathogen internalization resulting in caspase-1 processing and secretion of proinflammatory IL-1β (see Section 4.2). Dectin-1 is also known to influence the adaptive response to infection by encouraging Th1 and Th17 responses. This in turn may be important for the adjuvant-like activity of some dectin-1 ligands such as the β-1,3-glucan curdlan (see Section 5). Dectin-1 is critically important in establishing an effective antifungal response. Mice lacking Dectin-1 show increased susceptibility to fungal infections such as *Candida albicans*, *Pneumocystis carinii*, and *Aspergillus fumigatus*, which results from reduced production of protective cytokines and ROS.

2.2.4.2 Dectin-2 and Mincle

Like dectin-1, the ITAM-coupled receptors dectin-2 and mincle are most commonly expressed on a variety of myeloid cells. Both these receptors lack their own integral ITAM and therefore associate with the ITAM-containing FcRγ receptor to activate Syk, PKCδ, the CARD9 signalosome, the NLRP3 inflammasome, and stimulate the production of ROS. The repertoire of cytokines secreted following dectin-2 activation is more limited than after dectin-1 engagement.

Many of us will be familiar with the effects of dectin-2 activation as it is stimulated by house dust mite allergens and is therefore an important contributor to the immunopathology associated with dust mite allergy. A major component of the allergic response to dust mite allergens results from dectin-2–stimulated production of cysteinyl leukotrienes (Section 3.4.2). Dectin-2 is also activated in response to high mannose structures found on the cell wall of fungi such as *C. albicans* and *A. fumigatus*. Similarly, mincle also responds to fungi-related molecular patterns—in this case α-mannan on fungal cell walls—as well as endogenous ligands released from necrotic cells, and the mycobacterial cord factor trehalose 6,6′-dimycolate (TDM). Detection of TDM plays a central role in the identification and response to mycobacterial infection and subsequent proinflammatory cytokine secretion, nitric oxide production, and the stimulation of granuloma formation. The ability of mincle to detect TDM makes it a key PRR in the fight against tuberculosis infection, although there appear to be differences in the efficiency with which it can identify different mycobacterial strains. This may reflect differences in the precise molecular structure of TDM between strains, its release from the bacterium, or its accessibility to mincle. Regardless of why this difference in mincle activation occurs between strains, if researchers are able to pinpoint the functional basis of these differences, it may open new avenues for improving the efficacy of tuberculosis vaccines.

2.2.4.3 Tyrosine-Based Activation Motif–Independent Signaling by C-Type Lectin Receptorss

The classic example of ITAM-independent CLR signaling is provided by the DC-SIGN family of receptors, of which humans possess two, DC-SIGN and L-SIGN. These receptors are found on the surface of macrophages and DCs. Their ability to detect fucosylated and high mannose modified proteins shows that they are able to identify threats from all types of microorganisms. Activated DC-SIGN is rapidly endocytosed. This process allows DC-SIGN bound ligands to be subsequently presented to T cells. Although the engagement of DC-SIGN itself does not appear to directly lead to cytokine secretion, it does result in the modulation of other PRR signaling pathways. The precise functional impact on these pathways is dependent on the type of ligand detected by DC-SIGN. Mannose-modified ligand recognition leads to an increase in the transcription of IL-6, IL-10, and IL-12 expression following TLR4 activation, whereas fucosylated ligand detection results in the inhibition of IL-6 and IL-12 expression, but the enhancement of IL-10 production. Much of our understanding of DC-SIGN functionality and signaling stems from its importance as a receptor involved in the transfer of HIV-1 infection from DCs to T cells. This is facilitated by interactions between the gp120 component of the HIV-1 envelope protein and DC-SIGN.

2.2.4.4 C-Type Lectin Receptors Can Act as Inhibitory Receptors

The ITIM is an inhibitory signaling motif. The presence of an ITIM in the cytoplasmic tail of DCIR indicates that it can function as an inhibitory receptor.

This means that stimulation of DCIR should serve to limit and repress other PRR signaling pathways. However, this functionality seems to be limited to specific PRR pathways and hence DCIR activation does not initiate a generically immunosuppressive phenotype. For example, cytokine expression following TLR2, TLR3, and TLR4 stimulation is unaffected by simultaneous engagement of DCIR, whereas TLR9-dependent IFNα secretion and TLR8-dependent IL-12 and TNFα production are all downregulated by DCIR activation. This effect is believed to be the result of an effect upon tyrosine phosphorylation events within the cell, most likely mediated by the action of two tyrosine phosphatases, SHP-1 and SHP-2.

2.2.5 Cytoplasmic Pattern Recognition Receptors

It might be fair to say that the presence of PAMPs, DAMPs, or damage in the cytoplasm presents a potentially higher risk to the host, or at least the individual cell, than those that are extracellular or have been internalized as a result of pathogen/danger-mediated endocytosis. Consequently, it should be of no surprise that there are a diverse range of intracellular PRRs, whose role is to rapidly detect and respond to intracellular threats. As our understanding of the mechanisms involved in the cytoplasmic detection of cellular danger continues to improve, the repertoire of proteins and receptors involved in these pathways continues to expand. At the broadest level, these receptors can be broken down into two categories, those that detect nucleic acids, and those that do not. It is, however, more common to consider these receptors in the context of their actual signaling families, which is what shall be done here.

2.2.6 Nucleotide-Binding, Leucine-Rich Repeat-Containing Receptor Signaling

The NLR family are tripartite proteins that contain an N-terminal effector domain, a central NACHT domain within which is contained a nucleotide-binding domain, and a C-terminal leucine-rich repeat (Fig. 2.5). This domain organization shares strong parallels with the Resistance, or R proteins, which play a central role in the innate defenses of plants against pathogens. The NLRs are split into subfamilies based upon the identity of their N-terminal effector domains. The key subfamilies are the NLR family member with a CARD (NLRC) and NLR family member with a pyrin (NLRP).

A selection of the NLRs—NOD1, NOD2, NAIP, NLRC4, NLRP1, NLRP3—function as bona fide PRRs and activate an inflammatory immune response following detection of their activatory ligands. Others, such as NLRC5 and NLRP12, are also suggested to have PRR-related roles in the detection of viral and bacterial infections, respectively. NLRP6 is a crucial mediator of intestinal homeostasis and the maintenance of intestinal immunity. Commensal bacteria, especially segmented filamentous bacteria, are important for this functionality, but the exact mechanisms involved remain to be elucidated. NLRs also have a role to play in the transcriptional regulation of the MHC genes required for activation of the adaptive immune response. NLRC5 and CIITA control the expression of class I and class II MHC, respectively (see Section 5). NLRC3 negatively regulates inflammatory signaling through TLRs and STING, and NLRP4 has been associated with regulating autophagy. In a manner analogous to the Toll protein family in *Drosophila melanogaster*, a number of the *NLRP* genes appear to have roles in development, and polymorphisms in *NLRP7* are associated with the condition hydatidiform molar pregnancy.

For those NLRs that function as PRRs they, like the TLRs, use leucine-rich repeats to recognize the ligand. Until fairly recently it was unclear whether the NLRs bound their cognate ligands directly or indirectly. However, a series of biochemical studies have shown that, at least in the case of NOD1, NOD2, the NAIPs, and NLRX1, this interaction is direct and is predominantly mediated by the LRRs, although there are suggestions that the central NACHT region of the NAIPs and NOD2 may also contribute. What is clear is that the LRRs and the NACHT interact with one another to help control activation of the protein and that mutations that disrupt this interaction contribute to dysregulation of receptor signaling and autoinflammatory disorders.

2.2.6.1 NOD1 and NOD2 Receptor Signaling

NOD1 and NOD2 were the first NLRs to be described as PRRs. NOD1 shows a fairly ubiquitous pattern of expression, whereas NOD2 is more highly expressed in immune cells. They both are activated by pieces of peptidoglycan from the bacterial cell wall. NOD1 responds to γ-d-glutamyl-meso-diaminopimelic acid (iE-DAP), whereas the shorter fragment muramyl dipeptide (MDP) activates NOD2. Consequently, NOD2 responds to the presence of all bacteria, but NOD1 is specific for the detection of Gram-negative, and a few Gram-positive, bacteria. Activation results in proinflammatory cytokine production. NOD2 is activated by both the common *N*-acetyl form of MDP and the *N*-glycolyl form, which is found in *Mycobacteria* and the related *Actinomycetes*. The *N*-glycolyl–modified MDP is a more potent immune stimulus of NOD2 and various natural and synthetic analogs and derivatives of peptidoglycan have been shown to activate NOD2 with different levels of specificity. Factors that affect the activation of NOD2 include identity of the first two amino acids; presence and nature of amino acid modifications; length of the peptide stem; and the length and cleavability of the associated glycan sequence. NOD2 has also been reported to act as a sensor of viral infection through recognition of ssRNA, although this requires further validation as it would seem at odds with its role as a sensor of bacterial peptidoglycan.

Only a small number of bacterial infections lead to the presence of intracellular bacteria, and even fewer of these are found free in the cytoplasm. How then do NOD1 and NOD2 come into contact with their cognate ligands? It would appear that there are a wide variety of processes than can ultimately deliver peptidoglycan fragments into the cytoplasm leading to activation of NOD1 and

NOD2. These can include bacterial secretion systems, Gram-negative outer membrane vesicle shedding, autophagy, and specific import via peptide transporter channels such as solute carrier protein (SLC) 15A1 in the plasma membrane and SLC15A3 and 4 in the endosome membrane. Some bacteria, such as *Listeria monocytogenes*, modify their peptidoglycan to reduce its immunostimulatory potential.

NOD1 and NOD2 appear to recognize their ligands via their LRRs. Swapping the LRRs of NOD1 and NOD2 also switches their ligand specificity, and mutational disruption of the LRRs can often interfere with NOD1 and NOD2 function. Of course these mutations may interfere either with ligand recognition or the maintenance of an inactive conformation for the receptor. Retention of the autoinhibited conformation is further helped by interactions with chaperone proteins such as SGT1 (suppressor of G2 allele of Skp1), HSP70, and HSP90. The structure of NOD2 shows that LRR NACHT binding helps to stop NOD2 from being inappropriately activated. Disruption of receptor autoinhibition can lead to autoactivation of the receptor and the development of inflammatory conditions such as Blau syndrome. It is most likely that NOD1 and NOD2 bind their ligands directly, and there are biophysical studies using atomic force microscopy and surface plasmon resonance, which support this theory. NOD1 has been reported to respond to the activation of small GTPase proteins such as RhoA, RAC1, and CDC42 by bacterial effector proteins such as SopE from *Salmonella*. However, whether this occurs in addition to, in conjunction with, or instead of the direct detection of peptidoglycan is not yet clear.

The recognition of ligand by NOD1 and NOD2 may well be a dynamic process that also involves the binding of ATP, within the nucleotide-binding domain of the NACHT, to unlock the autoinhibited conformation of the receptor, freeing it to interact with its ligand and initiate signal transduction. Subsequent hydrolysis of ATP back to ADP allows the receptor to regain its autoinhibited form and may well work as a mechanism to either switch off NOD1 and NOD2 signaling, or at the very least minimize the chances of their inappropriate activation.

There is an increase in the levels of NOD1 and NOD2 at the plasma and endosomal membranes following receptor activation. However, it is as yet unclear whether this is the result of receptor migration post ligand detection or a recruitment process driven by the presence of ligand at these sites that then permits receptor activation. Once activated, the CARD of NOD1 and NOD2 interacts with the CARD of the adaptor protein RIPK2, an interaction likely to involve multiple interfaces on the respective CARDs. The precise interfaces used are, however, based on experimental observations likely to differ in their exact nature. This may be due in part to the fact that NOD2 possesses two CARDs whereas NOD1 has only one. It is currently unknown whether NOD1:RIPK2 or NOD2:RIPK2 forms any sort of large macromolecular complex analogous to the Myddosome or the inflammasome. RIPK2 also possesses a kinase domain and although originally described as a serine/threonine kinase, RIPK2 also functions as a tyrosine kinase. In fact autophosphorylation of Tyr474 within its own CARD appears to be important for regulating downstream proinflammatory signaling via NFκB and stress kinase pathways.

In addition to interacting with RIPK2, NOD2 can also interact with CARD9 in a process that specifically upregulates signaling via the stress kinase pathways. As yet, NOD1 has not been implicated in any CARD9-dependent signaling mechanisms. Despite the fact that both CARD9 and NOD2 have CARDs the interaction between the two proteins instead appears to be CARD independent and rely instead on regions of the NOD2 nucleotide-binding domain and the linker between the NOD2 CARDs and the NACHT domain.

2.2.6.2 Inflammasome-Based Signaling

Activation of the NLR proteins NLRP1, NLRP3, and NAIP/NLRC4 causes the formation of a large cytoplasmic multiprotein complex known as the inflammasome. NLRP6 and NLRP12 may potentially also form an inflammasome but this has not been conclusively proven. The primary function of the inflammasome is to induce the activation of the protease caspase-1 by facilitating the cleavage of its zymogen pro-caspase-1. Once activated, caspase-1 cleaves pro-IL-1β and pro-IL-18 to their active and proinflammatory forms, IL-1β and IL-18, ready for their release from the cell. Caspase-1 also cleaves the protein Gasdermin D, which then drives cell death by a process known as pyroptosis (Section 3.5.4).

Stimulation of inflammasome formation can be brought about by specific exogenous and endogenous ligands and disruption of cellular homeostasis. Inflammasome activators include ATP, potassium efflux, cholesterol crystals, silica, alum, uric acid, nucleic acids, membrane disruption, nigericin, flagellin, and anthrax lethal factor, to name but a few. There are many others and in fact the inflammasome itself can act as a danger signal following its release from dying cells. It is clear that NLRP1 and NAIP/NLRC4 respond to specific ligands, however, so many different molecules and processes activate the NLRP3 inflammasome that it is more accurate to view this complex as a sensor of homeostatic imbalance.

At the basic level the inflammasome is formed from a sensor protein (NLRP1, NLRP3, NAIP), an adaptor (ASC, NLRC4), and an effector caspase (caspase-1). However, it is clear that in the context of the rapid innate response to danger, the complex formed is heterogeneous and can contain multiple different sensors, adaptors, and caspases. Inflammasome formation is a rapid process, often occurring within minutes of stimulation and in the majority of cases only a single inflammasome is formed in each host cell. The final inflammasome complex can reach sizes of up to 1 micron in diameter, and can not only be of variable composition but also does not have a defined stoichiometry. The assembly process is dominated by protein:protein interactions, which can occur between sensor molecules, between sensors and adaptors, between adaptor proteins, between adaptors and effectors, and between effector caspases. Recent electron microscopy studies have indicated that the formation of filamentous protein structures is key to the overall assembly process, while superresolution microscopy of endogenous inflammasomes has suggested that the final global structure has a ring-like appearance.

Without doubt the inflammasome is a key protein complex in the innate immune proinflammatory response. A more comprehensive consideration of the mechanisms by which the inflammasome is activated to enable IL-1β production is given in Section 4.2, whereas Sections 4.3, 6.1, and 6.4 discuss the role of the inflammasome in *Salmonella* infection, cardiovascular disease, and autoinflammatory syndromes, respectively.

2.2.7 Nucleic Acid–Sensing Immune Receptors in the Cytoplasm

We have already seen that members of the TLR family, specifically TLRs 3, 7, 8, and 9, are able to sense the presence of foreign, or exogenously derived, nucleic acids in the endosome. This works well for responding to pathogenic threats that have been engulfed by the cell via endocytic and phagocytic pathways. But what happens with infections in the cytoplasm? How is this material sensed? It turns out that there is a wide range of nucleic acid–sensing PRRs within the cytoplasm that can detect and respond to various different forms of nucleic acid. The range, versatility, and redundancy displayed by these receptors strongly suggests that from a cellular perspective the presence of nonself, or inappropriate self, nucleic acid in the cytoplasm is indicative of a serious threat to the cell and potentially the organism and cannot be missed.

2.2.7.1 The RIG-I Family

The RIG-I family, a type of DExD/H box helicase, are the major sensors of cytosolic RNA. The family consists of three proteins, two of which—RIG-I and melanoma differentiation associated 5 (MDA5)—act as sensors to stimulate a protective immune response; while the third—laboratory of genetics and physiology 2 (LGP2)—acts as a negative regulator of inflammatory signaling. The ability of LGP2 to inhibit signaling stems from its lack of a CARD and therefore inability to propagate signal transduction. Activation of RIG-I and MDA5 can result in the induction of a range of inflammatory and immune signaling pathways. These include type I interferons via IRF activation and proinflammatory cytokines such as TNFα and IL-8 via stress kinase and canonical and noncanonical NFκB-mediated pathways. RIG-I is also able to stimulate caspase-1 activation and IL-1β and IL-18 production via a noncanonical inflammasome. A more detailed consideration of RIG-I–mediated signaling is provided in Section 4.4.3.

Unlike RIG-I, which preferentially binds to short dsRNA sequences with 5′-phosphates, MDA5 detects long pieces of dsRNA. This enables RIG-I and MDA5 to function in a broadly nonredundant manner in terms of their viral specificity, although there are viruses that both receptors recognize. However, broadly speaking, negative-sense RNA viruses activate the RIG-I–dependent pathway and positive-sense viruses turn on the MDA5 pathway. The CARDs of MDA5 and RIG-I interact with the CARDs of the adaptor protein MAVS to stimulate signal transduction.

2.2.7.2 The PYHIN Receptor Family

PYHIN proteins get their name from their possession of a PYD and a HIN200 domain. The PYD domain mediates signal transduction while the HIN200 binds to dsDNA through its OB folds. Most PYHIN proteins have just one HIN200 domain, although some, such as IFI16 in humans and IFI202 and IFI204 in mice, possess two. This usually results in a higher affinity for the binding of its dsDNA ligand. At least four confirmed PYHIN proteins exist in humans which include AIM2 and IFI16. Mice contain at least 11 PYHINs.

AIM2 signals via an inflammasome following recruitment of the key inflammasome adaptor protein ASC via PYD:PYD interactions and consequently activates caspase-1 leading to the release of IL-1β and IL-18. The mechanism of action of AIM2 is described in more detail in Section 4.2.1. IFI16 in contrast upregulates the production of type I interferons (see Section 3.1.3). From a mechanistic perspective the role of murine p202 is particularly interesting. p202 has two HIN200 domains and binds dsDNA in a manner very similar to that of AIM2. However, p202 does not have a PYD, or any other form of signaling effector domain, and therefore does not activate inflammatory signaling.

2.2.7.3 STING and the Innate Detection of Nucleic Acids

In addition to TLR9 in the endosome and the cytoplasmic AIM2, DNA can also be detected by a range of other PRRs. These include RNA Pol II, which creates dsRNA copies of poly(dA-dT) that subsequently activate RIG-I, as well as proteins such as Mre11, cGAS, DAI, DNA-PKcs, DDX41, and IFI16, all of which converge to activate the stimulator of interferon genes, STING (Fig. 2.12).

IFI16 is a member of the PYHIN family, like AIM2, and in addition to being able to activate the inflammasome to produce IL-1β and IL-18, IFI16 can also stimulate STING-dependent IFNβ production. IFI16 shuttles between the nucleus and the cytoplasm and detects foreign DNA in the nucleus and any form of DNA in the cytoplasm. Cytoplasmic levels of IFI16 increase under inflammatory conditions. DNA-PK and other members of the DNA damage response such as Mre11, Ku70, and Ku80 all appear to play a role in the induction of the interferon response to viral infection. In these cases STING appears to act as an adaptor protein in the induction of IFNβ.

DDX41, like the RIG-I like receptor (RLR) family, is a member of the DExD/H helicase family. It is not yet clear how many of the 60 or so family members have roles in nucleic acid detection. DDX41 is activated by interaction with cyclic dinucleotides such as cyclic di-GMP and cyclic di-AMP with a bacterial origin, where they are commonly used as signaling molecules. The role of DDX41 appears to increase the efficiency with which STING itself binds

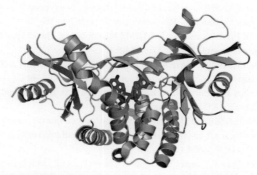

FIGURE 2.12   **Example structure of cytoplasmic nucleic acid–sensing pattern recognition receptors.** The closed complex structure formed by STING upon binding to cyclic dinucleotides, cGMP/cAMP (blue). The ligand fits into a pocket between the two STING chains that form the functional dimeric protein. Image generated from PDB 4LOI.

to, and is activated by, these cyclic dinucleotides. The enzyme cyclic GMP-AMP synthase has been shown to produce cyclic dinucleotides in response to cytoplasmic DNA, which then also act as a ligand for STING activation. Hence in these pathways, STING functions as a direct sensor of cyclic dinucleotides.

STING itself is a transmembrane protein that associates with the ER membrane. Its cytoplasmic domain exists as a v-shaped dimeric molecule in both the ligand-free and ligand-bound forms (Fig. 2.12). The conformation creates a large cleft in the molecule that acts as a binding site for a single cyclic dinucleotide resulting in a 2:1 receptor to ligand stoichiometry. Multiple interactions between the ligand and STING are made but binding does not change the nature of the dimer interface between the two protein molecules. Overall there is not a major change in STRING structure upon ligand binding with the exception of a loop between the second and third beta sheets, suggesting that this region may act as a molecular switch to stimulate subsequent signal transduction via TBK1 and IRF3 to activate IFNβ.

REFERENCES AND FURTHER READING

Section 2.1

Beyrau M, Bodkin JV, Noursharghar S. Neutrophil heterogeneity in health and disease: a revitalized avenue in inflammation and immunity. Open Biol November 21, 2012;2(11):120134.

Eberl G, Colonna M, Di Santo JP, McKenzie AN. Innate lymphoid cells: a new paradigm in immunology. Science 2015;348(6237):aaa6566.

Filep JG, Kebir DEl. Neutrophil apoptosis: a target for enhancing the resolution of inflammation. J Cell Biochem December 1, 2009;108(5):1039–46.

Geissmann F, Manz MG, Jung S, Sieweke MH, Merad M, Ley K. Development of monocytes, macrophages, and dendritic cells. Science February 5, 2010;327(5966):656–61.

Goldberg R, Prescott N, Lord GM, Macdonald TT, Powell N. The unusual suspects – innate lymphoid cells as novel therapeutic targets in IBD. Nat Rev Gastroenterol Hepatol 2015;12(5):271–83. Nature Publishing Group.

Gordon S, Plüddemann A, Martinez Estrada F. Macrophage heterogeneity in tissues: phenotypic diversity and functions. Immunol Rev November 2014;262(1):36–55.

Italiani P, Boraschi D. From monocytes to M1/M2 macrophages: phenotypical vs. functional differentiation. Front Immunol October 17, 2014;5.

Kadri N, Wagner AK, Ganesan S, Kärre K, Wickström S, Johansson MH, et al. Dynamic regulation of NK cell responsiveness. Curr Top Microbiol Immunol 2015:95–114.

Kolaczkowska E, Kubes P. Neutrophil recruitment and function in health and inflammation. Nat Rev Immunol February 25, 2013;13(3):159–75.

Merad M, Sathe P, Helft J, Miller J, Mortha A. The dendritic cell lineage: ontogeny and function of dendritic cells and their subsets in the steady state and the inflamed setting. Annu Rev Immunol March 21, 2013;31(1):563–604.

Miller JC, Brown BD, Shay T, Gautier EL, Jojic V, Cohain A, et al. Deciphering the transcriptional network of the dendritic cell lineage. Nat Immunol September 2012;13(9):888–99.

Novak ML, Koh TJ. Macrophage phenotypes during tissue repair. J Leukoc Biol June 1, 2013;93(6):875–81.

O'Sullivan TE, Sun JC, Lanier LL. Natural killer cell memory. Immunity October 2015;43(4):634–45.

Phillipson M, Kubes P. The neutrophil in vascular inflammation. Nat Med November 7, 2011;17(11):1381–90.

Pinegin B, Vorobjeva N, Pinegin V. Neutrophil extracellular traps and their role in the development of chronic inflammation and autoimmunity. Autoimmun Rev July 2015;14(7):633–40.

Reizis B. Regulation of plasmacytoid dendritic cell development. Curr Opin Immunol April 2010;22(2):206–11.

Reizis B, Bunin A, Ghosh HS, Lewis KL, Sisirak V. Plasmacytoid dendritic cells: recent progress and open questions. Annu Rev Immunol 2011;29:163–83.

Shifrin N, Raulet DH, Ardolino M. NK cell self tolerance, responsiveness and missing self recognition. Semin Immunol April 2014;26(2):138–44.

Sojka DK, Tian Z, Yokoyama WM. Tissue-resident natural killer cells and their potential diversity. Semin Immunol April 2014;26(2):127–31.

Vivier E, Tomasello E, Baratin M, Walzer T, Ugolini S. Functions of natural killer cells. Nat Immunol May 2008;9(5):503–10.

Wright HL, Moots RJ, Bucknall RC, Edwards SW. Neutrophil function in inflammation and inflammatory diseases. Rheumatology September 1, 2010;49(9):1618–31.

Section 2.2

Ahn J, Barber GN. Self-DNA, STING-dependent signaling and the origins of autoinflammatory disease. Curr Opin Immunol December 2014;31:121–6.

Berke IC, Li Y, Modis Y. Structural basis of innate immune recognition of viral RNA. Cell Microbiol March 2013;15(3):386–94.

Boyle JP, Parkhouse R, Monie TP. Insights into the molecular basis of the NOD2 signalling pathway. Open Biol December 2014;4(12). pii:140178.

Brubaker SW, Bonham KS, Zanoni I, Kagan JC. Innate immune pattern recognition: a cell biological perspective. Annu Rev Immunol March 21, 2015;33(1):257–90.

Bryant CE, Orr S, Ferguson B, Symmons MF, Boyle JP, Monie TP. International union of basic and clinical pharmacology. XCVI. Pattern recognition receptors in health and disease. Pharmacol Rev 2015;67(2):462–504.

Burdette DL, Vance RE. STING and the innate immune response to nucleic acids in the cytosol. Nat Immunol December 14, 2012;14(1):19–26.

Connolly DJ, Bowie AG. The emerging role of human PYHIN proteins in innate immunity: implications for health and disease. Biochem Pharmacol December 2014;92(3):405–14.

Davis BK, Wen H, Ting JP-Y. The inflammasome NLRs in immunity, inflammation, and associated diseases. Annu Rev Immunol April 23, 2011;29:707–35.

Fütterer K, Wong J, Grucza RA, Chan AC, Waksman G. Structural basis for syk tyrosine kinase ubiquity in signal transduction pathways revealed by the crystal structure of its regulatory SH2 domains bound to a dually phosphorylated ITAM peptide. J Mol Biol August 1998;281(3):523–37.

Gao P, Ascano M, Zillinger T, Wang W, Dai P, Serganov AA, et al. Structure-function analysis of STING activation by c[G(2′,5′)pA(3′,5′)p] and targeting by antiviral DMXAA. Cell August 2013;154(4):748–62.

Gay NJ, Gangloff M, O'Neill LA. What the Myddosome structure tells us about the initiation of innate immunity. Trends Immunol March 2011;32(3):104–9. Elsevier Ltd.

Gay NJ, Symmons MF, Gangloff M, Bryant CE. Assembly and localization of Toll-like receptor signalling complexes. Nat Rev Immunol 2014;14(8):546–58.

Jounai N, Kobiyama K, Shiina M, Ogata K, Ishii KJ, Takeshita F. NLRP4 negatively regulates autophagic processes through an association with beclin1. J Immunol February 1, 2011;186(3):1646–55.

Kagan JC. Signaling organelles of the innate immune system. Cell December 2012;151(6):1168–78.

Kagan JC, Magupalli VG, Wu H. SMOCs: supramolecular organizing centres that control innate immunity. Nat Rev Immunol October 31, 2014;14(12):821–6. Nature Publishing Group.

Kawai T, Akira S. Toll-like receptors and their crosstalk with other innate receptors in infection and immunity. Immunity 2011;34(5):637–50.

Keestra AM, Winter MG, Auburger JJ, Frässle SP, Xavier MN, Winter SE, et al. Manipulation of small Rho GTPases is a pathogen-induced process detected by NOD1. Nature April 11, 2013;496(7444):233–7.

Lamkanfi M, Dixit VM. Mechanisms and functions of inflammasomes. Cell May 22, 2014;157(5):1013–22. Elsevier Inc.

Lemos H, Huang L, McGaha TL, Mellor AL. Cytosolic DNA sensing via the stimulator of interferon genes adaptor: Yin and Yang of immune responses to DNA. Eur J Immunol October 2014;44(10):2847–53.

Lin SC, Lo YC, Wu H. Helical assembly in the MyD88-IRAK4-IRAK2 complex in TLR/IL-1R signalling. Nature 2010;465(7300):885–90.

Loo Y-M, Gale M. Immune signaling by RIG-I-like receptors. Immunity May 27, 2011;34(5):680–92. Elsevier Inc.

Monie TP. NLR activation takes a direct route. Trends Biochem Sci March 2013;38(3):131–9. Elsevier Ltd.

Motta V, Soares F, Sun T, Philpott DJ. NOD-like receptors: versatile cytosolic sentinels. Physiol Rev January 1, 2015;95(1):149–78.

Reikine S, Nguyen JB, Modis Y. Pattern recognition and signaling mechanisms of RIG-I and MDA5. Front Immunol 2014;5:342.

Rock KL, Latz E, Ontiveros F, Kono H. The sterile inflammatory response. Annu Rev Immunol January 2010;28:321–42.

Schattgen SA, Fitzgerald KA. The PYHIN protein family as mediators of host defenses. Immunol Rev September 2011;243(1):109–18.

Schroder K, Tschopp J. The inflammasomes. Cell March 19, 2010;140(6):821–32.

Shang G, Zhu D, Li N, Zhang J, Zhu C, Lu D, et al. Crystal structures of STING protein reveal basis for recognition of cyclic di-GMP. Nat Struct Mol Biol July 24, 2012;19(7):725–7. Nature Publishing Group.

Singer H, Biswas A, Nuesgen N, Oldenburg J, El-Maarri O. NLRP7, involved in hydatidiform molar pregnancy (HYDM1), interacts with the transcriptional repressor ZBTB16. PLoS One June 29, 2015;10(6):e0130416. Oudejans C, editor.

Song DH, Lee JO. Sensing of microbial molecular patterns by Toll-like receptors. Immunol Rev 2012;250(1):216–29.

Thépaut M, Guzzi C, Sutkeviciute I, Sattin S, Ribeiro-Viana R, Varga N, et al. Structure of a glycomimetic ligand in the carbohydrate recognition domain of C-type lectin DC-SIGN. Structural requirements for selectivity and ligand design. J Am Chem Soc February 20, 2013;135(7):2518–29.

Unterholzner L. The interferon response to intracellular DNA: why so many receptors?. Immunobiology November 29, 2013;218(11):1312–21. Elsevier GmbH.

Yin Q, Fu T-M, Li J, Wu H. Structural biology of innate immunity. Annu Rev Immunol March 21, 2015;33(1):393–416.

Section 3

Effector Mechanisms and Cellular Outputs

3.1 CYTOKINES

Cytokines are small proteins of usually not more than 20 kDa in size, which act as the primary effector molecules of the innate immune response. They are produced and secreted primarily from immune cells in response to the detection of danger and damage and are therefore often the result of pattern recognition receptor (PRR)-mediated signaling. Nonimmune cells can also secrete cytokines, particularly under inflammatory conditions. Cytokines provide a method of communication not only between different cells at the site of infection, damage, or inflammation but also to other distal parts of the body—i.e., they are intercellular messengers. They provide specific instructions to both immune and nonimmune cells and dictate the nature, precise form, and the duration of the innate inflammatory response. Cytokines can take the form of growth factors, be either proinflammatory or antiinflammatory, be potentially damaging and protective, act locally and systemically, act as chemoattractants (chemokines), alter cellular functionality, drive processes such as hematopoiesis, enable the innate and adaptive responses to interface with one another, and are a major immunopathological mediator.

The nomenclature of cytokines is diverse and in many cases they are still referred to by their historical names rather than the officially accepted nomenclature. Specific subgroups of cytokines exist and these include chemokines—cytokines that act as chemoattractants for other cells; lymphokines—cytokines secreted by lymphocytes; and interleukins—leukocyte-secreted cytokines that function on other leukocytes. However, these descriptions are not necessarily entirely accurate as many nonleukocyte cells also respond to interleukins. Cytokines are also often grouped on the basis of their functional properties, and throughout the biomedical literature, one will find reference to proinflammatory and antiinflammatory cytokines, as well as to type 1 and type 2 cytokines. Type 1 and type 2 cytokines generally refer to those secreted by Th1 and Th2 cells, respectively (Fig. 3.1).

In this section, I will begin by briefly introducing the main properties and functions of the key groups of cytokines associated with the innate immune response. Where appropriate, these have been grouped by family to keep

The Innate Immune System. http://dx.doi.org/10.1016/B978-0-12-804464-3.00003-X

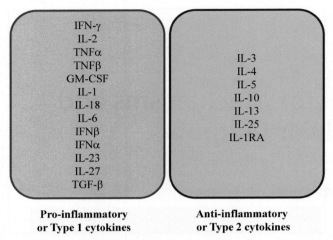

IFN-γ	
IL-2	
TNFα	
TNFβ	IL-3
GM-CSF	IL-4
IL-1	IL-5
IL-18	IL-10
IL-6	IL-13
IFNβ	IL-25
IFNα	IL-1RA
IL-23	
IL-27	
TGF-β	
Pro-inflammatory	**Anti-inflammatory**
or Type 1 cytokines	**or Type 2 cytokines**

FIGURE 3.1 **Example groupings of major immune cytokines.** The major inflammatory cytokines have been grouped into the two most common delineations encountered—proinflammatory and/or type 1 cytokines, or antiinflammatory and/or type 2 cytokines. The precise function or impact of an individual cytokine often depends on what other cytokines are also being expressed.

similar cytokines together. Space dictates that these descriptions cannot be completely comprehensive, but the references and further suggested reading at the end of the section provides resources from which more detailed information can be obtained. This is then be followed by descriptions of some of the other key innate immune effector mechanisms such as the acute phase response, eicosanoids, the complement and coagulation cascades, reactive oxygen species (ROS), and cell death.

3.1.1 The Interleukin-1 Family

Interleukin is one of the most important inflammatory mediators and is intimately connected to acute and chronic inflammatory processes. It is a core contributor to the pathogenesis of most inflammatory conditions and is a common therapeutic target for the treatment of chronic inflammation. Within the interleukin-1 cytokine family, there are 11 members—seven cytokines that act as proinflammatory agonists (IL-1α, IL-1β, IL-18, IL-33, IL-36α, IL-36β, IL-36γ), one antiinflammatory cytokine (IL-37), and three receptor antagonists (IL-1Ra, IL-36Ra, IL-38). The receptor family for the IL-1 cytokines (the IL-1R family) also contains 11 members. These receptors are located in the plasma membrane and contain a mix of activating, regulating, and decoy receptors. They are formed from three extracellular immunoglobulin-like folds and an intracellular Toll/interleukin-1 resistance (TIR) signaling domain, with the exception of SIGRR and IL-18BP, which only contain one immunoglobulin-like fold.

Interleukin-1: IL-1 itself has two biological forms IL-1α and IL-1β. These are encoded from different genes and lack significant homology but both signal via the IL-1R1 receptors. They are pyrogenic and act upon almost all cell types to stimulate the production of proinflammatory cytokines. IL-1α is synthesized by many different tissues, but especially by those found in the epithelial surfaces and in organs such as the liver and spleen that have higher chance of pathogen contact and damage. IL-1α is produced in an active form and kept in storage vesicles ready for release upon the recognition of danger, damage, or cell death. At this point, it can immediately initiate signaling to recruit inflammatory cells and mediators. In contrast, IL-1β is produced as an inactive precursor protein that requires processing to an active form before its release from the cell. The main, but not the only, mechanism by which pro-IL-1β is activated is through caspase-1–mediated cleavage following inflammasome activation (see Section 4.2). Because of its highly inflammatory nature, inhibition of IL-1 signaling, for example, through the administration of anti-IL-1 biologics such as anakinra is a common therapeutic approach for the treatment of chronic inflammatory conditions (see Section 6).

Engagement of IL-1 with IL-1R1 (Fig. 3.2) results in receptor heterodimerization, recruitment of the adaptor protein MyD88 to the intracellular TIR domain, and the activation of a signaling cascade very similar to that seen with Toll-like receptors (TLRs). This process involves formation of the multiprotein complex Myddosome following the recruitment of IRAK proteins and the ultimate activation of NFκB and stress kinase signaling pathways.

Interleukin-18: Just like IL-1β, IL-18 (Fig. 3.2) is also translated into an inactive pro form, pro-IL-18, which is processed by caspase-1 following inflammasome activation. IL-18 is important for the activation of natural killer (NK) cells and in promoting a Th1 immune response. It promotes IFNγ secretion through its stimulation of lymphocytes and stimulates macrophages to secrete TNFα. IL-18 has been associated with a wide range of chronic inflammatory conditions including metabolic syndrome, psoriasis, and inflammatory bowel disease. The action of IL-18 can be limited by the antagonistic activity of the decoy receptor IL-18BP, which binds to the active form of IL-18 and serves to limit its inflammatory potential. Under homeostatic conditions IL-18 appears to be particularly important for the maintenance of the integrity of the intestinal barrier, production of some antimicrobial peptides, and the regulation of the commensal flora. Disruption of IL-18 function leads to alterations in the make up of the intestinal microflora. However, during inflammation it appears that IL-18 can actually make a disease worse by interfering with the function of goblet cells and the production of mucus.

Interleukin-33 and -36: IL-33 interacts with the ST2 receptor and is an important cytokine in pushing the immune response away from a Th1-dominated profile and toward a Th2 response. Meanwhile, the different IL-36 molecules favor a Th1 or Th17 biased immune response and generally mirror

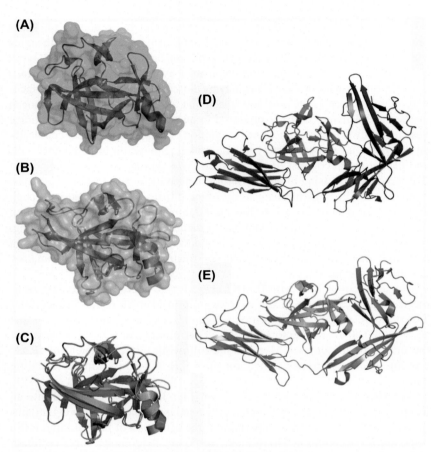

FIGURE 3.2 The structure of IL-1β and IL-18. The three-dimensional structure of two of the major proinflammatory cytokines (A) IL-1β (PDB 1I1B) and (B) IL-18 (PDB 3WO2) are presented as a cartoon and surface representation. (C) An overlay of IL-1β (red) and IL-18 (orange) highlights the similarity in the global structure of these two cytokines. Complexes of (D) IL-1β (PDB 4DEP) and (E) IL-18 (3WO3) with their respective receptors, IL-1R1 and IL-18R1, indicate that the mode of binding for both these ligand–receptor interactions is highly similar. Panels A, B, and C are orientated the same as one another, whereas panels D and E have the same orientation as each other.

the activities of IL-1 albeit at a more sedate level. The IL-36 cytokines do not undergo caspase-mediated processing, but if processing is artificially induced, then they become much more proinflammatory.

The antagonists—IL-1Ra, IL-36Ra, IL-37, and IL-38: The proinflammatory nature of IL-1 signaling makes it essential that the process is properly regulated. This occurs at many different levels, one of which is through the use of antagonists that interfere with the cognate receptor ligand interactions. IL-1Ra and IL-36Ra interfere with the interactions between IL-1 and the IL-1R and between IL-36 and the Il-36R, respectively. IL-37 on the other hand appears to bind to the IL-18R and downregulate inflammation through an SIGRR-dependent mechanism. The absence of IL-37 results in a two- to threefold increase in the inflammatory response to bacterial lipopolysaccharide (LPS). IL-38 shares around 40% homology with both IL-1Ra and IL-36Ra proteins and appears to block binding to both IL-1R and IL-36R, but much less effectively than the primary antagonists for these receptors do.

3.1.2 The Tumor Necrosis Factor Families

There are two superfamilies of tumor necrosis factor (TNF)-related proteins, the TNF superfamily and the TNFR superfamily. The former describes the ligands and the latter the plasma membrane–bound receptors and each family contains a functionally diverse range of proteins. Both superfamilies have strong structural identity—the ligands form trimeric complexes and the receptors possess cysteine-rich ectodomains. There are three different categories of TNFR—(1) decoy receptors that lack a cytoplasmic signaling domain; (2) DD-containing receptors; and (3) TRAF-engaging receptors. TNF-related signaling is integral to many types of cell–cell communication and is relevant for processes relating to inflammation and immunity, cell death, organ and tissue development, and cellular homeostasis.

The variety of contributions to immune function from TNF family members at both the adaptive and innate level is diverse. This relates to the fact that despite their structural conservation, TNF family members share little similarity in their surface residues. Various receptor ligand combinations (CD40:CD40L, Fas:FasL, TNF:TNFR1/2) act as initiators of the extrinsic pathway of apoptosis, some (OX40:OX40L) are involved in T-cell responses, and others (TNFα:TNFR1/2, LTα:TNFR1) are critical for the innate proinflammatory response to infection. TNFα (Fig. 3.3) is highly proinflammatory and an important component of both the acute and chronic inflammatory responses. This has resulted in anti-TNF biologics being commonly used to treat chronic inflammatory conditions such as inflammatory bowel disease. The interaction of TNFα with TNFR2 (Fig. 3.3) leads to signaling via NFκB-mediated pathways and is generally viewed to be prosurvival in nature. These signaling pathways are dependent on the involvement of the E3 ubiquitin ligases TRAF2 and TRAF3. In contrast, engagement of TNFR1 instead results in the recruitment of TRADD to the TNFR1 DD and initiates cell death pathways that may result in either apoptotic or necroptotic cell death (Section 3.5). The same cell death pathways are also activated by LTα:TNFR1 engagement.

3.1.3 The Interferon Family

Interferons can be split into three subsets—type I, II, and III interferons. The type I interferons contain IFN-α, -β, -ε, -κ, and -ω; the type II interferons consist solely of IFNγ; and the type III interferons contain IFNλ1, 2, 3, and 4. From an immunological perspective the most important, and certainly

(A)

(B)

(C)

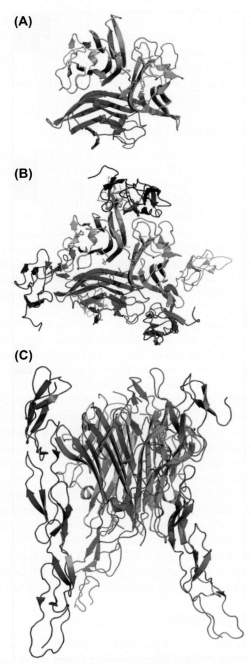

FIGURE 3.3 Example structures of TNF and the TNF-TNFR2 complex. (A) The trimeric form of the proinflammatory cytokine TNF (PDB 1TNF) with each subunit colored separately. (B) Top view of the complex between TNF and the TNFR2 receptor (PDB 3ALQ). The complex consists of a TNF trimer and three TNFR2 molecules. The orientation and coloring of the TNF molecules is the same as in panel A. (C) A side view of the TNF:TNFR2 complex.

the best studied, interferons are IFNα, IFNβ, and IFNγ. The type I interferon IFNβ is secreted from, and acts upon, almost all cell types, while IFNα and the type II interferon, IFNγ, although active on most, if not all cell types, are mainly produced from immune cells, with plasmacytoid dendritic cells representing a major source of both IFNα and IFNγ in response to viral infection.

The production and secretion of type I interferons is stimulated by the activation of a range of different PRRs following the activation of the transcription factors IRF3 and IRF7. These include TLR3, 4, 7, 8 and 9, RIG-I, LRRFIP1, RNAPolIII, and multiple intracellular DNA sensors such as IFI16, DAI, and DNA-PK, all of which seem to function via the protein STING (see also Section 2.2.7.3). Following secretion, type I interferons interact with the heterodimeric receptor interferon alpha receptor (IFNAR) (Fig. 3.4), which results in activation of the JAK/STAT signaling pathway. The same pathway is also activated by IFNγ, albeit through the engagement of the IFNGR protein and recruitment of JAK1 and JAK2 as opposed to JAK1 and TYK2. Together these events result in the activation of interferon-stimulated genes (ISGs) such as PKR, OAS1, MX1, ADAR, and APOBEC3G among others. The function of these ISGs is to drive the antiviral immune response and create an environment within the stimulated cell that is nonpermissive for viral replication. This helps to limit the spread and damage associated with the infection. The deaminase APOBEC3G has been shown to play a particularly important role in the restriction of HIV-1 infection.

IFNγ (Fig. 3.4) is a highly proinflammatory cytokine. This is primarily due to its ability to increase leukocyte recruitment, enhance phagocytosis, upregulate major histocompatibility complex (MHC) expression, and dramatically enhance the cytolytic activity of macrophages and NK cells. Activation of macrophages with IFNγ is a key element in driving the destruction of phagocytosed microbes and in inhibiting and combating intracellular infection of the macrophages themselves. IFNγ along with TNFα is a key driver of macrophage activation into a classical proinflammatory, or M1, phenotype. Activated NK cells are key producers of IFNγ early in the immune response, although γδ T cells also contribute. During the later stages of the immune response, T cells become more important contributors to its synthesis. IFNγ has been associated with the progression of various autoinflammatory disorders including rheumatoid arthritis and type 1 diabetes.

3.1.4 Interleukin-6 and Interleukin-8

IL-6 is produced by many cells and particularly macrophages, fibroblasts, and T cells. It is multifunctional and acts on a wide variety of cell types. For example, it stimulates hepatocytes to produce acute phase proteins and acts on leukocytes to direct their trafficking in response to inflammation. It also influences the wider immune response and contributes to hematopoiesis. An important role of

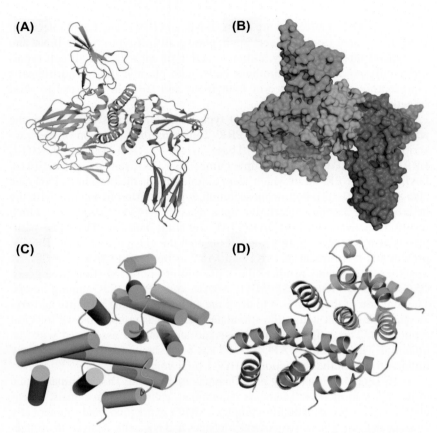

FIGURE 3.4 **The structure of Type I and II interferons.** (A) Cartoon and (B) surface representations of the type I interferon IFNα2 (cyan) in a ternary complex with its receptor interferon alpha receptor 1 (IFNAR1) (green) and IFNAR2 (magenta) (PDB 3SE3). IFNα2 has a helical structure and bridges between the two receptors. The membrane would be positioned at the bottom of the image. Sixteen type I interferons signal through the IFNARs but with different physiological responses that stem, at least in part, from the manner in which the Type I IFN interacts with IFNAR. (C) and (D) Cylindrical and cartoon images of the bovine IFNγ dimer (PDB 1D9G). The two monomers are colored cyan and green. Rather unusually this dimer is created through the swapping of helices between the two monomers to create an intertwined structure rather than simply possessing a dimer interface.

IL-6 is the induction of fever. Although weakly pyrogenic in its own context, Il-6 can enter the systemic circulation and contribute to the production of the highly pyrogenic prostaglandin E2.

IL-8 is a great example of a cytokine with chemotactic properties—i.e., a chemokine. It is one of the major chemokines involved, if not the major one, in the recruitment of neutrophils to the site of inflammation or infection. The official nomenclature form chemokines splits them into groups based on the position of key cysteine residues in their structures. By far the most common

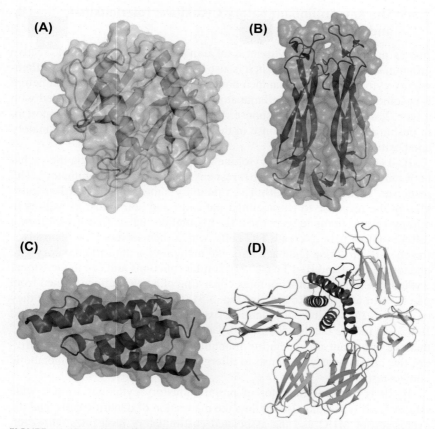

FIGURE 3.5   **Example structures from the interleukin family.** Cartoon and surface representations of: (A) human IL-8 (PDB 1IL8), which forms from an antiparallel beta-sheet and two alpha helices; (B) the dimeric human IL-17 (PDB 4HR9); (C) human IL-4 (PDB 2B8U), a mainly helical cytokine that forms a complex with a heterodimer of the IL4Rα (cyan); and IL-13Rα1 (green) as shown in panel (D) (PDB 3BPN).

groupings are denoted with the prefixes CXC and CC, with CXCL and CXCR referring to a ligand and a receptor, respectively. Many chemokines are known by the official nomenclature, but some such as IL-8 (CXCL8) have generally retained their traditional names. Chemokines are crucial in the maintenance of immune cell homeostasis and the recruitment and migration of immune cells to sites of need.

IL-8 (Fig. 3.5) is secreted by PRR-activated macrophages and damaged and PRR-activated endothelium. It is also secreted in response to proinflammatory cytokines. This helps ensure rapid and timely recruitment of effector cells, particularly neutrophils. Recruited and activated neutrophils act as a further source of IL-8 secretion. IL-8 interacts with the receptors CXCR1 and CXCR2.

3.1.5 The Key Antiinflammatory Cytokines: Interleukin-4, -5, -10, and -13

Just as proinflammatory cytokines are important for driving the protective inflammatory response of a host, it is also important for there to be antiinflammatory cytokines that can dampen down and switch off inflammation before it becomes damaging. Antiinflammatory cytokines are often associated with a type 2, or Th2, immune response. IL-4, -5, -10 and -13 are all important in pushing the immune response in the direction of a Th2 antiinflammatory composition.

IL-4 (Fig. 3.5) is the main cytokine responsible for promoting the switch between a proinflammatory Th1 response and an antiinflammatory Th2 response. Its association with Th2 immunity shows that it is a key cytokine in the response to extracellular parasites and helminths, as well as in allergy-related immune responses. IL-4 stimulates naive T cells to follow a differentiation path to create Th2 cells, which then secrete IL-4 themselves to generate a positive feedback loop and maintain the antiinflammatory Th2 phenotype. IL-4 and IL-13 have very similar functions and can in fact signal through the same receptor complex consisting of a heterodimer formed from one IL-4Rα and IL-13Rα1 chain (Fig. 3.5). This is despite the fact that they only share 25% amino acid identity. Exposure of macrophages to IL-4 and IL-13 can induce the development of "alternatively activated macrophages" that are important for mediating immunity to helminth infection, for driving the inflammatory response to allergens, and in maintaining metabolic homeostasis.

IL-10 is a potent inhibitor of proinflammatory cytokines from a wide range of cell types and also inhibits the maturation of dendritic cells, and the expression of MHC and the associated costimulatory molecules. However, IL-10 does stimulate the differentiation of mast cells and B cells. IL-10 forms a high-affinity interaction with its heterodimeric receptor on the surface of target cells and signals via JAK/STAT pathways. Disruption of IL-10 signaling results in the development of severe, often chronic, inflammation. Although in the short term, IL-10 neutralization can improve the clearance of viral infections.

3.1.6 The Interleukin-17 Family, Interleukin-21, and Interleukin-22

The IL-17 family of cytokines is important in the regulation of both innate and adaptive host defenses and inflammation. In conjunction with IL-21 and IL-22, they are critical to the development of the Th17 subset of T cells. There are six members of the IL-17 family, but most of our functional understanding relates to the two most closely related members IL-17A (Fig. 3.5), which is usually called just IL-17, and IL-17F. IL-17A and F are proinflammatory, have broadly redundant functions, and are principally produced by

Th17 cells. γδ T cells also secrete IL-17 in response to bacterial infection of the epithelial or mucosal surface. IL-17A and IL-17F are important for the protective response against fungal pathogens such as *Pneumocystis carinii* and *Candida albicans*.

IL-17A and IL-17F are recognized by a heterodimeric complex formed from two receptor chains—IL-17RA and IL-17RC. IL-17A binds with higher affinity to IL-17RA, while IL-17F has a stronger affinity for IL-17RC. The receptor complex is found on the plasma membrane of a variety of cell types including macrophages, fibroblasts, neutrophils, and epithelial cells. Engagement of the receptor complex by either IL-17A or IL-17F results in the activation of classical proinflammatory cytokines via NFκB and MAPK signaling pathways. These then recruit inflammatory cells such as macrophages and neutrophils to the site of infection. In addition to being important in fungal and surface bacterial infections IL-17, cytokines also play a key role in the pathogenesis of various chronic inflammatory conditions such as rheumatoid arthritis, multiple sclerosis and inflammatory bowel disease.

IL-21 and IL-22 are also both related to Th17 T cells. IL-21 is structurally homologous to IL-2, -4, and -15 and is secreted by NK cells and T cells, especially the Th17 CD4$^+$ T cell subset. Exposure to IL-21 activates the JAK/STAT signaling pathway and results in an increase in NK cell and CD8 T cell cytotoxicity and also influences B-cell development. IL-21 appears to be activatory for most cell types that it interacts with; however, it serves to inhibit the maturation of dendritic cells.

Il-22 is also expressed by NK cells and activated T cells. It undergoes extensive glycosylation and signals through a heterodimer of the IL-10 and IL-22 receptors, with the IL-22R component determining cell specificity. Like many interleukins, IL-22 functions through the JAK/STAT pathway. IL-22 expression is upregulated by bacterial expression and IL-22 signaling is particularly important for the activation of antimicrobial genes in keratinocytes. This is consistent with the increased bacterial burden and intestinal damage observed for IL-22 knock out mice on infection with *Citrobacter rodentium*.

3.1.7 Additional Immune-Related Cytokines

The range and diversity of the cytokines and their contribution to innate immunity goes beyond the current scope of this work. However, there are a few other cytokines that merit brief mention in the context of their immune roles.

The growth factor granulocyte-macrophage colony-stimulating factor (GM-CSF) is responsible for the differentiation of progenitor cells in the bone marrow into the respective cell types. Its production, from a broad range of immune and nonimmune cells, is stimulated by danger-mediated PRR activation thereby enabling rapid expansion of the cell types required to combat the threat of damage or infection. The secreted GM-CSF cytokine interacts with a surface receptor formed from a heterodimer of GM-CSFRα, which provides low-affinity binding, and GM-CSFRβ, which mediates signal transduction and the activation of JAK-STAT–based signaling pathways. The importance of macrophages in chronic inflammatory diseases makes disruption of GM-CSF production or signaling a potential therapeutic target.

The chemokine monocyte chemoattractant protein 1 (MCP1; CCL2) shows a large increase in expression and secretion during inflammation. It forms concentration gradients via interaction with glycosaminoglycans present on cell surfaces and free in solution. These gradients enable MCP1 to recruit monocytes to the site of damage via interaction with the receptor CCR2. Interestingly, MCP1 appears to be able to perturb the integrity of the blood–brain barrier (BBB) and contribute to the passage of cells across the BBB, which may contribute to the pathogenesis of some infections of the central nervous system.

Macrophage inflammatory protein (MIP) 1α (CCL3) and MIP-1β (CCL4) are closely related chemokines secreted from activated macrophages, and most other hematopoietic cells, which signal via CCR5, one of the major coreceptors for HIV infection. As with many secreted cytokines and chemokines, both proteins are translated with a signal peptide that is removed as part of the secretory process. They appear to exist as a dimeric molecule but are highly prone to aggregate in a concentration-dependent, dynamic, and reversible manner. They are important in maintaining the recruitment and activation of immune cells during the inflammatory response. They also stimulate the release of histamine from basophils and eosinophils. Excessive or prolonged MIP production has been associated with a range of chronic inflammatory conditions throughout the body including osteoarthritis, multiple sclerosis, atopic dermatitis, and ulcerative colitis.

The transforming growth factor beta (TGFβ) proteins are part of a family of cytokines that have wide-ranging roles in the control of cellular functions such as proliferation, migration, adhesion, cytokine secretion, repair, fibrosis, and differentiation. TGFβ is usually stored and secreted in a latent form that can be activated by a variety of methods, but most of them appear to involve binding to integrins. It has a wide range of immune functions, some of which are context dependent. TGFβ acts as chemoattractant for monocytes and also, at high concentrations, stimulates IL-1β production. It also promotes leukocyte infiltration into tissues, stimulates the secretion of some cytokines such as the MIPs and MCP1, and through suppression of T cell function can inhibit T-cell–driven cytokine secretion.

3.2 ACUTE PHASE PROTEINS AND THE ACUTE PHASE RESPONSE

The acute phase response is an innate inflammatory reaction that occurs at a systemic level in response to homeostatic disruption within the host. This disruption can have many causes, which include infection, tissue injury or trauma, cancer, or immunological dysfunction. It is mediated by a wide range of proteins found in the plasma, known as acute phase proteins. To be classed as an acute phase protein the circulating level of the protein needs to either increase, or decrease, by at least 25% from their steady-state level. Because of the sensitivity of acute phase proteins to the homeostatic balance of the host, their concentrations are commonly used as markers of health and disease.

The induction of the acute phase response is often triggered by the local production of cytokines, which themselves are being produced following local infection or injury. As such the detection of danger/damage-associated molecular patterns (DAMPs) and pathogen-associated molecular patterns (PAMPs) by PRRs is a crucial step in the initiation of the acute phase response. The activation of inflammatory cells and the vascular system leads to the further production of more inflammatory cytokines, which can then migrate into the circulation and initiate systemic changes. Particularly important for this process are TNFα, IL-1, and IL-6, with IL-6 playing a major role in the systemic changes. The major physiological and systemic changes associated with the acute phase response include the induction of fever, reduced leukocyte number in the blood, complement activation, upregulation of the blood coagulation system, increased glucocorticoid levels, loss of appetite, alterations in serum mineral levels, and changes in the concentrations of acute phase proteins.

Most acute phase proteins are produced in the liver, and this becomes a site of rapid protein synthesis following the cytokine-driven initiation of the acute phase response. IL-6 is particularly potent at stimulating hepatocytes to synthesize acute phase proteins. Major acute phase proteins that increase in concentration include C-reactive protein, serum amyloid A, haptoglobin, and fibronectin. In some instances the increase in concentration of C-reactive protein and serum amyloid A can be more than 1000-fold. For those acute phase proteins such as albumin and transferrin, which show a drop in concentration, the rate of their synthesis falls (Fig. 3.6).

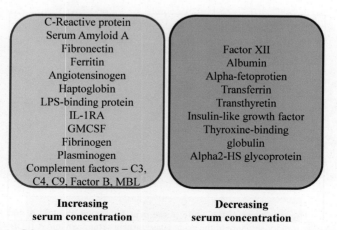

C-Reactive protein	
Serum Amyloid A	Factor XII
Fibronectin	Albumin
Ferritin	Alpha-fetoprotien
Angiotensinogen	Transferrin
Haptoglobin	Transthyretin
LPS-binding protein	Insulin-like growth factor
IL-1RA	Thyroxine-binding
GMCSF	globulin
Fibrinogen	Alpha2-HS glycoprotein
Plasminogen	
Complement factors – C3,	
C4, C9, Factor B, MBL	
Increasing	**Decreasing**
serum concentration	**serum concentration**

FIGURE 3.6 **Selected acute phase proteins.** Proteins on the left hand side increase in concentration in the acute phase response, whereas those on the right hand side decrease in concentration. This list is only a selection of the acute phase proteins.

C-reactive protein is an example of a short pentraxin and functions in a manner analogous to classical PRRs. It exists in a ringlike disc conformation formed from five copies of the 25 kDa monomeric protein (Fig. 3.7) and recognizes phosphocholine that is released from dying cells and also present on the surface of some microorganisms. This can facilitate complement activation and stimulate phagocytic clearance of dying cells and danger threats. While some of the effect of C-reactive protein is proinflammatory, there is also plenty of evidence that it can interfere with the interaction of neutrophils with the endothelium and therefore behave in an antiinflammatory manner.

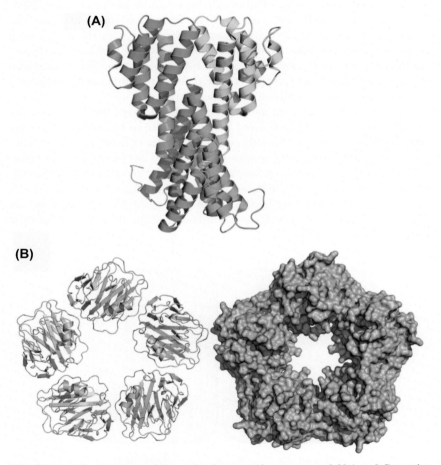

FIGURE 3.7 **The structures of the acute phase proteins serum amyloid A and C-reactive protein.** (A) The tertiary structure of the acute phase protein serum amyloid A (PDB 4IP8). Each monomer in the complex is presented in a different color. The fibrillar structure has the potential to aggregate further. (B) C-reactive protein exists as a pentameric porelike protein that can interact with phosphocholine (PDB 1GNH).

Serum amyloid A forms a helical structure and functions as a hexamer (Fig. 3.7). Its primary role appears to be to bind to high-density lipoprotein particles in the circulation. It is a proinflammatory molecule that acts as an attractant for both neutrophils and mast cells, and itself stimulates proinflammatory cytokine synthesis as a result of interactions with cell surface receptors such as the PRRs TLR2 and TLR4, scavenger receptors such as CD36, and through activation of the NLRP3 inflammasome. As well as functioning as an acute phase protein serum amyloid A is also a possible candidate molecule for driving the pathogenesis of a number of chronic inflammatory conditions including amyloidosis, atherosclerosis, and rheumatoid arthritis.

3.3 REACTIVE OXYGEN SPECIES

At the basic level, ROS is the term used to describe any free radical or reactive molecule that is derived from molecular oxygen. It includes species such as peroxides, superoxides, hydroxyl radicals and ions, and nitric oxide. In most cases ROS are produced as a result of aerobic respiration in the mitochondria, or through the action of oxidoreductase enzymes. ROS are high-energy, highly reactive molecules and have the potential to cause significant levels of cellular damage if not tightly controlled. The cell therefore invests significant levels of resource into the production of both enzymatic and nonenzymatic approaches to neutralize unwanted ROS. For example, the glutathione antioxidant system serves not only to neutralize ROS such as peroxides, but is also important in the regeneration of other antioxidant molecules. The destructive potential of ROS does, however, make these molecules excellent for the killing of microorganisms, and they consequently play an important role in the host defense against infection and are key components of phagocytic cell functions. In fact, the "oxidative burst" employed by phagocytic cells to mediate the breakdown and destruction of pathogens results from the deliberate production of ROS through the action of specific enzymes such as NADPH oxidase. ROS also has other functions aside from those involving pathogen killing. For example, ROS can function in both intracellular and extracellular signaling pathways and is also important in the control of gene expression and the induction of apoptosis. ROS have also been strongly linked to activation of the NLRP3 inflammasome, although the precise mechanism by which they might achieve this remains enigmatic (see Section 4.2).

Nitric oxide, which only has a half-life of around 4 s, is a particularly interesting ROS as it has two different methods of synthesis, which reflect different functional roles. Nitric oxide synthase produces nitric oxide via the oxidation of L-arginine. One form of the enzyme is constitutively active and produces low levels of nitric oxide in neuronal and endothelial cells, which then functions in a signaling capacity to increase levels of cGMP. The physiological effects of this signaling activity are seen through the relaxation of the vasculature, interference with the aggregation of platelets, and for neuronal cells, mediation of neuronal transmission. In contrast, cells that wish to use nitric oxide as a defense mechanism, which includes macrophages, fibroblasts, and hepatocytes, use an inducible form of nitric oxide synthase. This leads to much higher levels of nitric oxide production compatible with a role in host defense. The expression levels of inducible nitric oxide synthase are regulated by inflammatory stimuli and cytokines thereby ensuring that these higher levels of nitric oxide production only occur when physiologically necessary.

3.4 ENZYMATIC CASCADES AND ENZYMATIC ACTIVATION

3.4.1 Blood Coagulation Pathways

The blood coagulation system is an important part of the innate defense against infection. By restoring the integrity of the vasculature, it acts as a physical block to the further entry of pathogens and many of the stimuli that activate an innate inflammatory response also serve to activate coagulation. In many ways, inflammation and coagulation simply represent different arms of the protective response to cellular damage and infection. In fact one view is that the vertebrate coagulation system is evolutionarily evolved from the innate immune system.

The process of coagulation is driven by the activity of specific serine proteases, which are rapidly activated at the local level. These proteases work to produce thrombin, which drives the conversion of fibrinogen to fibrin. The key host factor that triggers activation of the coagulation cascade is the transmembrane protein Tissue Factor. Tissue Factor is expressed on the surface of cells in close proximity to the vessel wall, but not on the surface of the endothelial cells lining the vessel wall, which are in constant contact with the blood. As soon as the vessel wall is damaged, which might be the result of infection, trauma, or cell death, the Tissue Factor is exposed to the circulating blood and immediately interacts with Factor VII, which is present in the blood. This causes the activity of Factor VII to increase by more than a 1000-fold, which enables it to cleave and activate Factor X. This combined approach of spatial segregation followed by a binding-induced increase in proteolytic activity is a critical element in limiting the inappropriate activation of the coagulation cascade—which would obviously have potentially disastrous effects. Once activated, Factor X is able to convert prothrombin to thrombin, which then ultimately leads to the localized generation of a fibrin clot from fibrinogen.

Excessive coagulation is harmful. As such, the production and activity of thrombin is tightly regulated. One form of regulation occurs through the action of anticoagulates such as heparin-antithrombin and the protein C thrombomodulin system. Decreased levels of antithrombin are seen with sepsis. Protein C thrombomodulin is broadly antiinflammatory as it decreases secretion of proinflammatory cytokines from monocytes, inhibits neutrophil chemotaxis, and reduces leukocyte recruitment by downregulating adhesion molecules.

3.4.2 Eicosanoids

The classical inflammatory responses of fever, pain, and swelling are often brought under control through the administration of "painkillers" such as aspirin and other nonsteroidal antiinflammatories. A significant part of the success of these medications results from their ability to interfere with and block pathways involved in the biosynthesis of metabolically active inflammatory lipids, such as the eicosanoids, prostaglandins, and leukotrienes. Many of these nonsteroidal antiinflammatories work by interfering with cyclooxygenase (COX) 1 and COX2 signaling, which subsequently stops a large proportion of the ongoing synthesis of bioactive lipids.

Biochemically, eicosanoids can be described as bioactive lipids derived from arachidonic acid and other polyunsaturated fatty acids with a 20-carbon chain length. Functionally, eicosanoids contribute to a wide range of inflammatory and homeostatic signaling pathways. The contribution of the eicosanoids to the proinflammatory response has long been recognized. However, it is becoming increasingly apparent that this is an oversimplification and that certain eicosanoids can also induce an antiinflammatory state and contribute to the resolution of inflammation. Part of this increased understanding and awareness has resulted from the development of metabolomics, particularly lipidomics, and the associated improvements in both the diversity of lipid molecules that can be detected by mass spectrometry–based approaches, and the sensitivity with which these molecules can be found.

Eicosanoids involved in inflammation are predominantly produced by COX-mediated oxidation of polyunsaturated fatty acids, although the lipoxygenase (LOX) pathway has also been shown to be activated during inflammation. In fact LOX-derived eicosanoids play a particularly important role in the process of bronchoconstriction and the specific recruitment of leukocytes to sites of damaged tissue. Eicosanoids can also be produced by nonenzymatic free radical pathways and the action of cytochrome P450 enzymes. These pathways seem to be either less important for inflammation or are simply less well understood in this context.

It is important to realize that the actual pattern of eicosanoids produced in response to cellular danger, cellular damage, or infection is highly variable. It depends heavily on the precise cell types involved and their actual location within the host tissues. For example, even when stimulated in exactly the same manner, not all macrophages will produce the same spectrum, or indeed the same quantities, of eicosanoids; the precise outputs will depend on their originating tissue type. The biological activity of eicosanoids is also affected by tissue type and not all eicosanoids produce the same effect on different tissue or cell types. Prostaglandin E_2 induces pain and inflammation in neurons and acts through a G-protein coupled receptor (GPCR) signaling pathway. However, in macrophages it appears that prostaglandin E_2 has antiinflammatory properties as a result of reducing TNF levels and increasing IL10 production.

Almost all eicosanoid biosynthetic pathways require arachidonic acid, or other polyunsaturated fats, to be available in their free form. However, the cell normally stores these molecules in an esterified form. To become available for eicosanoid biosynthesis, these essential precursor molecules require deesterification to increase the concentration of the free forms of the fatty acids. In most cells this role is performed by phospholipase A2. The intracellular levels of various functional forms of phospholipase A2 are increased in response to immune receptor activation, such as occurs via TLRs and other PRRs. This therefore allows an immediate increase in eicosanoid production in response to cellular danger. This response can, however, lead to the production of what is known as an "eicosanoid storm," which refers to the rapid, large-scale production of proinflammatory eicosanoids. If this "storm" is not tightly regulated, it can have potentially devastating, even fatal, effects. However, when under proper control, elements of the "eicosanoid storm" are actually believed to provide an important functional role in the initiation of the process of postinflammation resolution. In fact the parallel activation of TLR and inflammasome signaling seems to result in the simultaneous activation of classical inflammatory pathways via NFκB and IL-1β signaling, along with an eicosanoid-driven resolution-primed pathway.

3.4.3 Complement

The complement system has been briefly introduced in Section 1.3.4.2. Here I will provide an overview of the activation and regulation of the three pathways along with a brief discussion of the pathological and immunological activity.

3.4.3.1 Activation of the Complement Cascade

The three activation systems of the complement system are known as the alternative pathway, the lectin pathway, and the classical pathway. Although they are each activated in distinct manners, these pathways ultimately converge with the same effector mechanisms following the formation of a multiprotein complex known as the C3 convertase.

The alternative pathway: The first of these pathways to be activated, whether as a result of the presence of pathogens or because of homeostatic disruption, is the alternative pathway (Fig. 3.8). This is because, at least in healthy hosts, the alternative pathway continually functions with a low level of constitutive activity. This constitutive activity is the result of spontaneous hydrolysis of the labile thioester bond in the complement protein C3 resulting in the production of two fragments known as C3a and C3b. The rate at which this hydrolysis occurs can be increased by the interaction of C3 with a variety of biological, or synthetic, surfaces. Importantly these surfaces often take the form of pathogen membranes. Once generated, C3b interacts with exposed hydroxyl groups, which because of the short half-life of C3b of approximately 60 μs, must occur close to the site of initial C3b production. C3b that binds to the surface of host

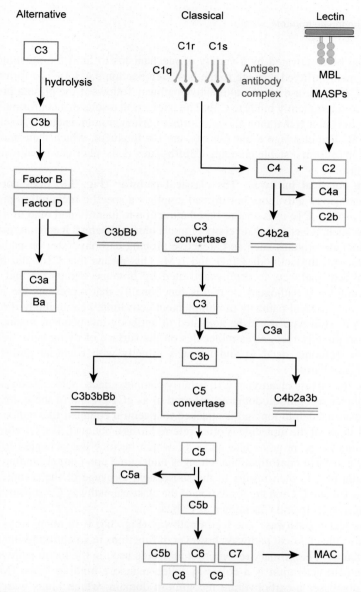

FIGURE 3.8 A brief schematic of the three pathways of complement activation. The alternative pathway begins with the autohydrolysis of C3 and the cleavage of Factor B by Factor D to generate Bb. The C3 convertase forms at the target surface by the interaction of C3b and Bb. This allows rapid generation of more C3b, the release of C3a, which then acts as a chemoattractant and an anaphylatoxin, and leads to the formation of the C5 convertase (C3b3bBb), following the recruitment of more C3b molecules. In the classical pathway recognition of antigen-antibody complexes by C1q, C1r and C1s stimulate cleavage of C4 and C2 to create the C4b2a C3 convertase molecule. The identity of the C3 convertase is the same for the lectin pathway but here cleavage of C4 and C2 occurs following binding of pathogen sugars by mannose-binding lectin (MBL) and MBL-associated serine protease (MASP) proteins. In both the classical and lectin pathways the further recruitment of C3b molecules to the C3 convertase leads to the production of a C5 convertase of the composition C4b2a3b. The C5 convertases cleave C5 releasing C5a to act as an anaphylatoxin and chemoattractant and enabling C5b to initiate formation of the membrane attack complex (MAC) via recruitment of C6, C7, C8, and C9.

cells can be inactivated by a variety of mechanisms to limit the potential for complement-inflicted damage to the host (see Section 3.4.3.3). The formation of the C3 convertase via the alternative pathway follows if the plasma protein Factor B subsequently binds to C3b. The interaction results in a conformational change in Factor B that then allows a further plasma protein, Factor D, to cleave Factor B. The cleavage event releases the Bb fragment, which then interacts with C3b to form a stable complex C3bBb—this is the alternative pathway C3 convertase.

The classical pathway: The classical pathway (Fig. 3.8) does not rely on spontaneous activation, but instead employs a specific recognition protein known as C1q. C1q uses charge-based attraction to identify and bind to its targets. As such, it has a wide diversity of molecules with which it can interact and these include proteins such as C-reactive protein, carbohydrates on pathogen surfaces, and the antibodies IgG and IgM. This means that C1q, and hence the classical pathway, is readily activated by immune complexes and antibody-complexed pathogens. It is this functionality that represents the major role of the classical pathway of complement activation, i.e., antibody-directed activation. However, it can be activated in antibody-independent manners as C1q also directly recognizes molecules on the surface of dying cells, various DAMPs including dsDNA, and interacts directly with bacterial porins and lipopolysaccharide.

The spatial organization of C1q is fairly complex. Each molecule consists of six globular recognition domains, referred to as gC1q. Each of these domains complexes a calcium ion and is attached to a central collagen-like region. The overall shape of the molecule is often referred to as a bouquet. The C1 complex also contains the proteins C1s and C1r, which become autoactivated following the extensive conformational changes undergone upon target binding. The activation of C1s then results in the subsequent cleavage of the complement proteins C4 and C2 and the formation of the classical pathway C3 convertase— a complex of C4b and C2a known as C4b2a.

The lectin pathway: The lectin pathway (Fig. 3.8) is in many ways very similar to the classical pathway; however, it functions in an antibody-independent manner. The primary recognition molecule used in the lectin pathway of complement activation is a collectin called mannose-binding lectin (MBL). MBL possesses a carbohydrate recognition domain, which binds with relatively low affinity to carbohydrates, such as mannose, N-acetyl glucosamine, and fucose, which are commonly found on microbial surfaces. It does not bind to sialic acid, which is the most common terminal sugar found in vertebrates. This contributes to the specificity of the lectin pathway for pathogens. To compensate for the low binding affinity of the individual carbohydrate recognition domains in MBL, the protein forms multimers and is therefore able to make multiple interactions with its target surface resulting in high-avidity interaction. In humans MBL is usually present in the plasma as an oligomer formed from three to six trimers. The other proteins that can activate the lectin pathway are all examples of ficolins. In humans these are known as L-ficolin, H-ficolin, and M-ficolin. Both L-ficolin and H-ficolin are synthesized by the liver, but M-ficolin is produced in the blood and also by the lungs. These ficolins are broadly similar to MBL and also form oligomeric complexes of trimeric bundles. As such, they also use low-affinity, high-avidity interactions with their targets. However, unlike MBL the ficolins employ a fibronectin domain and not a carbohydrate recognition domain to interact with their target. This results in a different repertoire of molecular targets. L-ficolin and M-ficolin are specific for acetylated sugars, including lipoteichoic acid, which is a major component of the Gram-positive bacterial cell wall. H-ficolin binds to galactose and D-fucose.

Carbohydrate binding by MBL and the ficolins is not to lead to the formation of the C3 convertase required to initiate complement effector functions. For this to happen, MBL and the ficolins activate the MBL-associated serine proteases MASP-1 and MASP-2. The initial interaction with MASP-1 and MASP-2 occurs in the plasma before target binding. At this point both the proteases are present as inactive zymogens; however, carbohydrate binding causes conformational changes that result in activation of the proteases. The activated MASP-1 and MASP-2 proteases can then proceed to cleave C2 and C4 and, in a manner analogous to the classical pathway, results in the formation of the C3 convertase C4b2a.

To reiterate, the key process in complement activation is the formation of the C3 convertase. This is the point at which each pathway converges and without the C3 convertase the downstream effector functions of the complement system cannot be initiated. The multiprotein C3 convertase complex produced by the classical and lectin pathways is identical, having the form C4b2a. In contrast, the alternative pathway results in the formation of a C3 convertase from fragments of C3 and Factor B, to give a complex of C3bBb.

3.4.3.2 The Effector Mechanisms—Inflammation, Killing, and Phagocytosis

Convergence of the three complement activation pathways occurs at the level of formation of the C3 convertase complex, whether this is in the form C4b2a or C3bBb. From this point on the potential effector, mechanisms are shared and can be broken down into three main processes, which include the following:

1. The promotion of inflammation and phagocyte recruitment,
2. Direct killing via the formation of a membrane attack complex (MAC), and
3. Stimulation of target (i.e., pathogen) phagocytosis.

The promotion of inflammation and phagocyte recruitment: The continual recruitment of immune cells, particularly phagocytic ones such as macrophages and neutrophils, and the associated inflammation is driven by the complement components C3a and C5a. Because of their inflammatory properties, both of these molecules are known as anaphylatoxins. Given their proinflammatory properties the overproduction of anaphylatoxins can lead to the induction of anaphylactic shock, which is very similar in manifestation to sepsis.

C3a and C5a form small bundles of three to four helices and activate immune cells by interacting with the GPCRs C3aR and C5aR. It is not just phagocytic cells that are influenced by the complement anaphylatoxins; they actually modulate a wide range of immune cells. For example, they can trigger the release of histamines from mast cells and basophils; C3a activates B cells and triggers IL-10 secretion from T-cells, while C5a induces Erk signaling and drives a Th1 adaptive response (see Section 5). It also appears that C3a has some antiinflammatory behavior as it appears to be able to inhibit neutrophil degranulation. C5a is a more potent anaphylatoxin than C3a, and C4a also appears capable of functioning in a similar manner, but with a much lower level of activity.

Direct killing via the formation of a MAC: The direct killing of pathogens by complement is driven by the formation of a pore-forming multiprotein structure known as the MAC. The MAC creates a pore, about 10 nanometers across, in the target membrane leading to osmotic dysregulation and cell death. The formation of the MAC begins with the generation of the C5 convertase complex. This happens when additional C3b fragments are recruited to and interact with the C3 convertase. This can occur with either form of the C3 convertase and results in the formation of the following complexes—C4b2a3b and C3bBb3b—the latter complex is sometimes referred to as $C3b_2Bb$. The formation of the C5 convertase is a rapid process. This is primarily because of the high concentration of C3, which is the most abundant complement protein in the plasma, and serves as a ready source of C3b, following its spontaneous hydrolysis during activation of the alternative pathway. This ensures a steady supply of C3b around the C3 convertase, and it has been estimated that each C3 convertase complex has approximately 1000 C3b molecules in close proximity.

The role of the C5 convertase is to mediate cleavage of C5 to C5a and C5b. As described previously, C5a functions as an anaphylatoxin. C5b on the other hand undergoes extensive conformational change that allows it to interact with C6. This serves to further the recruitment of C7, C8, and C9, which interact with one another in an irreversible manner to form a porelike structure. Attraction to the target membrane is driven by the lipophilic properties of C5b, C6, and C7, whereas C8 is principally responsible for penetrating and permeabilizing the membrane. The final pore can contain between 2 and 18 C9 molecules.

The MAC does not work well against Gram-positive bacteria as their cell wall is too thick. However, it is highly efficient at killing Gram-negative bacteria and lysing erythrocytes—other host cells, which are metabolically active, tend to be resistant to MAC-driven lysis. The MAC induces cell lysis in a multihit fashion, in which any one individual pore is insufficient to cause lysis, but as MAC number increases, cellular dysfunction also increases before reaching a point where pore number is sufficient to cause lytic death. The importance of the MAC in the defense against Gram-negative bacteria is most clearly seen in relation to *Neisseria meningitidis* infection. Individuals with defects, usually of genetic origin, in their MAC have shown heightened susceptibility to recurrent infections.

Stimulation of target (i.e., pathogen) phagocytosis: Complement-mediated stimulation of phagocytosis results from the fact that many complement components, and particularly C3b, are powerful opsonins. One could argue that enhancing phagocytosis is in fact the primary role of complement activation in the innate immune repertoire. An extremely important point to be aware of here is that complement-driven opsonization enables phagocytosis of pathogens long before the induction of the adaptive response and the generation of antibodies, which of course are also important mediators of phagocytosis. This has two main benefits. In the first instance it encourages the early clearance of pathogens before they have the chance to cause damage or disease. Secondly, phagocytosis of pathogens and their subsequent breakdown allows the presentation of antigens via antigen-presenting cells in a manner that will prime and drive the adaptive immune response.

The key complement opsonins are fragments of the C3 molecule. These are recognized by specific complement receptors (CR1, CR2, CR3, CR4, and CRIg), which are themselves expressed on the surface of a variety of cell types. CR1 is found on phagocytic cells and erythrocytes; CR2 on B cells; CR3 and CR4 on monocytes, with enhanced levels on macrophages; and CRIg is found at high levels on macrophages. Within the macrophage population, Kupffer cells display particularly high levels of CR3 and CRIg, which helps to explain the efficiency with which these cells can remove immune complexes and pathogens from the blood.

3.4.3.3 Regulating the Complement Cascade

It should be obvious from the methods of activation and the effector mechanisms described earlier that proper regulation of the complement cascade is paramount. Without this the host is in serious threat of extensive complement-mediated damage or even death. Consequently, there are a wide range of regulatory processes and proteins whose role is to ensure that the induction of the complement system occurs in a controlled and beneficial manner.

There are multiple distinct mechanisms by which complement pathway activation can be regulated. For example, the classical pathway is inhibited by the presence of heme and proteoglycans such as chondroitin-4 sulfate, which are often released from dying cells and bind to and inhibit C1q. Other members of the C1 complex, C1s and C1r, are targeted and inactivated by the C1 inhibitor (C1inh) protein leading to their dissociation from the complex. C1inh is also able to limit the activity of the MASP-1 and MASP-2 proteases needed in the lectin pathway. Further regulation of the lectin pathway occurs through the action of homologues to MASP-1 and MASP-2. Proteins such as MASP-3,

Mapp4, and Map19, are able to bind to MBL and the folicins in the place of MASP-1 and MASP-2 and subsequently inhibit the downstream cleavage of C2 and C4, thereby stopping formation of the C3 convertase.

Further regulation of the activation of the complement cascades and the formation of the C3 convertase is provided in the form of a number of proteins found both in the plasma and on the membrane of host cells. These include Factor H, Factor I, decay accelerating factor, CR1, and also membrane cofactor protein (MCP). Factor I, CR1, and MCP can function together to stimulate proteolysis of C4b and C3b thereby inhibiting C3 convertase formation at the membrane or stimulating its breakdown. Factor H is particularly important for regulation of the alternative pathway and is often viewed as a master regulator of C3b. Factor H is able to bind free C3b—it actively competes with Factor B—in the plasma and therefore stops it acting either as an opsonin or becoming part of the C3 convertase. Factor H is also able to bind to the C3 convertase and stimulate the release of the Bb fragment, which serves to inactivate the complex. The dissociation of membrane-bound C3 convertase complexes by Factor H is helped by the ability of Factor H to interact with glycosaminoglycans on the cell surface. Consequently, increase in the expression levels of glycosaminoglycans on cell surfaces leads to enhanced recruitment of Factor H and a concomitant reduction in complement activation, especially of the alternative pathway. Binding to C3b also serves to limit the formation of the C5 convertase. Additional mechanisms for limiting formation of the classical and lectin pathway C3 convertase also exist and include the activity of the C4 binding protein (C4BP). C4BP is able to drive the dissociation of the C4b2a C3 convertase complex and also functions as a cofactor for the inactivation of C4b by Factor I.

The MAC is also subject to regulation and again there are multiple pathways that function to achieve downregulation of MAC activity. For example, the plasma proteins clusterin and vitronectin scavenge components of the MAC from the plasma and therefore stop complex formation. Should a MAC be formed on a host cell, then the majority of cells have good surface expression levels of the MAC regulator CD59. CD59 is a glycosylphosphatidylinositol-anchored receptor that interacts with the MAC and stops it from being able to permeabilize the membrane. MACs can also be lost from host cells through the process of membrane shedding and exocytosis or the process of membrane internalization and subsequent degradation of the MAC components.

3.4.3.4 Complement and Disease

Inappropriate and excessive activation of the complement system can inflict damage upon the host and in the most severe cases may induce anaphylactic shock and possibly even death. These effects do not result from any specific defect in the complement system, but are because of overstimulation or overactivation. However, the large number of proteins involved in the complement system shows that there are many different points at which problems can occur.

Sometimes these are the result of deficiencies in specific complement proteins and factors. A common side effect of such deficiencies is an increased susceptibility to recurrent bacterial infections and an increased severity of infection. Complement deficiencies have also been linked with a number of specific conditions and diseases.

Defects in the activation, or the regulation, of the classical pathway are linked closely with problems in clearing dead or dying cells and immune complexes from the circulation. This has been associated with the development of conditions such as rheumatoid arthritis and systemic lupus erythematosus (SLE). The most common deficiency in the Caucasian population is depletion of the Factor C2, which occurs in between 1 in 10,000 and 1 in 20,000 individuals. This deficiency is also more commonly associated with SLE patients. In children, C2 deficiency can lead to an increased frequency of colds and ear infections. Defects or mutations in the regulatory protein Factor H can lead to the formation of the severe, but rare, kidney disorder atypical hemolytic uremic syndrome.

3.4.4 Caspases

Caspases are cysteine proteases that play a crucial function in many cell death and inflammatory pathways such as apoptosis (Section 3.5.1), necroptosis (Section 3.5.3), pyroptosis (Section 3.5.4), inflammasome signaling, and IL-1 mediated inflammation (Section 4.2). Broadly speaking, caspases have historically been split into two functional groups—those involved in apoptosis and those involved in inflammation. In humans, apoptotic caspases include caspase-2, caspase-3, caspase-6, caspase-7, caspase-8, caspase-9, and caspase-10; whereas the inflammatory caspases are traditionally described as caspase-1, caspase-4, caspase-5, and caspase-12. Mice do not possess the genes for caspase-4 and caspase-5, but instead produce a single orthologous protein known as caspase-11. As much of our understanding of caspase function has come from murine studies, a large proportion of the recent published literature on inflammatory caspases focuses on caspase-11. Some, maybe even most of, the functionality attributed to caspase-11 can, however, also be attributed to either, or sometimes both, caspase-4 and caspase-5 in humans.

As our understanding of caspase function, cell death pathways, and inflammatory signaling has improved, it has become clear that to simply classify caspases as apoptotic or inflammatory is a major oversimplification. For example, caspase-8 is involved in activation of cell death via extrinsic pathways, which can result in either apoptosis of necroptosis. Caspase-8 is also involved in a wide range of inflammatory signaling mechanisms including both canonical and noncanonical inflammasome pathways and the induction and processing of IL-1β in a Fas-mediated manner. Caspase-1 has also been shown to not only be a key enzyme in the processing of proinflammatory cytokines such as pro-IL1β and pro-IL18, but also drives pyroptotic cell death through cleavage of the cytosolic protein Gasdermin D, a process also mediated by caspase-11 and caspase-4 (Section 3.5.4).

Because of their potent enzymatic activity and the potentially dangerous consequences of the inappropriate activation of cell death and inflammatory signaling, all caspases are synthesized as zymogens—an inactive precursor that requires specific activation. When present as a zymogen, i.e., inactive, caspases are known as pro-caspases. Pro-caspases consist of an N-terminal region containing a prodomain and a C-terminal catalytic domain formed from a large and small subunit. The prodomains vary both in size and composition. Effector or executioner caspases that function late in cell death pathways, such as caspase-3, possess short unstructured prodomains. In contrast, initiator caspases that act earlier in the signaling of cell death, as well as inflammatory caspases, contain structured prodomains from the death domain superfamily of protein structures. These are either caspase recruitment domains (CARDs) or death effector domains and facilitate the interaction of the pro-caspase with other protein partners in the assembly of macromolecular signaling complexes that help facilitate caspase activation, such as the inflammasome. Activation of the pro-caspase often occurs through autocatalytic cleavage mediated by the induced proximity of separate pro-caspases. In the case of effector caspases in the cell death pathways, this cleavage is often mediated by the upstream initiator caspases. Whereas, the initiator and inflammatory caspases often perform autocatalytic cleavage, having been brought close enough together. Once activated, all caspases appear to function as heterodimers containing two copies of the C-terminal large and small catalytic subunits.

The active sites of caspases are highly similar to one another and use a catalytic cysteine residue. They have a general target consensus sequence of DXXD-A/G/S/T (positions known as P4,P3,P2,P1-P1′), with the site of cleavage marked by a hyphen. Within this consensus the first position, the P4 position, is generally aspartic acid, D, in caspase-3 and caspase-7, but for the inflammatory caspases is usually a larger residue such as tryptophan or tyrosine. All caspases have a very strong preference for an aspartic acid residue in the P1 position. Similarly, they all prefer a small amino acid in the P1′ site immediately after the point of cleavage. Therefore, while each caspase has its own preferred primary cleavage sequence, they are generally able to cleave a range of actual sequences, albeit with varying or reduced efficacy. This explains why pan-caspase inhibitors that interfere with a broad range of, or even all, caspases are readily available for research into caspase function. It also means that inhibitors that are reported to be specific for a particular caspase may actually show off-target effects. Hence, as with many pharmacological approaches, one must interpret data about caspase function obtained using caspase inhibitors carefully because it may not just be the targeted caspase that is being affected. Given that over 1500 known caspase substrates exist in the human proteome, the potential for wider and unexpected effects on cell function to occur is not insignificant.

The inflammatory caspases, specifically caspase-1, caspase-4, and caspase-5 in humans, and caspase-1 and caspase-11 in mice, are key contributors to inflammasome-mediated inflammatory signaling, via the processing of pro-IL1β and pro-IL18, and cell death via pyroptosis. These areas have been discussed in more detail in Sections 3.5.4 and 4.2. Caspase-12 on the other hand may well have an antiinflammatory role and is thought to limit caspase-1–mediated inflammation in mice. Almost all humans, with the exception of around 20% of populations of African descent, encode for a variant of caspase-12 that contains a polymorphism in exon 4 of the *CASP12* gene. This polymorphism introduces a premature stop codon and leads to the translation of a truncated protein containing the N-terminal CARD domain, but not the catalytic subunits. This truncated version is known as caspase-12S and is believed to help provide protection against excessive inflammatory responses to bacterial infection, particularly those by Gram-negative bacteria, by reducing the likelihood of these infections leading to septic shock. It is therefore plausible that the polymorphism arose as a protective phenotype against an excessive and therefore dangerous inflammatory response to bacterial infection.

3.5 CELL DEATH

Cell death is a natural process that is central to homeostatic maintenance and the natural turnover of cell populations; it is also intrinsically connected to the response to cellular danger. It represents a path of last resort for a cell that has either been irreparably damaged or is unable to control an infection. Its importance as a defense mechanism is underpinned by the wide-ranging approaches adopted by pathogens, or indeed tumor cells, to avoid cell death. Poxviruses encode for many proteins that interfere with cell-death pathways. For example, CrmA is a viral protein produced by members of the *Orthopoxvirus* genus, which includes variola virus, the cause of smallpox, and vaccinia virus, which was used in vaccines to eradicate smallpox. CrmA interferes with the function of both caspase-1 and caspase-8 and therefore inhibits cell death via pyroptosis, necroptosis, and apoptosis. Of course some infections, such as those caused by poliovirus, deliberately cause cell lysis as a mechanism for enabling further spread and dissemination.

Cell death can be a deliberate choice by the cell, induced in a controlled manner by death-inducing stimuli, or be accidental. All of these scenarios occur in the case of cell death associated with inflammatory and immune responses. The following sections provide an overview of apoptotic, necrotic, necroptotic, and pyroptotic cell death from the perspective of the innate immune and inflammatory responses to cellular danger. They do not, however, delve into the full complexities and molecular details of these processes, which could easily fill a textbook in their own right.

3.5.1 Apoptosis

Apoptosis defines a process of tightly regulated and controlled cell death with distinct morphological changes and is often referred to as programmed cell death. It is automatically switched on in the absence of prosurvival factors and signals. The morphological changes include condensation of the chromatin, fragmentation of the DNA, fragmentation of the nucleus, cell shrinkage and detachment from neighboring cells, plasma membrane blebbing, and aggregation of cytoplasmic filaments. These changes are macroscopically visible. Importantly, cellular contents are not released into the extracellular environment during apoptosis, and the dying cell is rapidly phagocytosed by macrophages. This results in a lack of inflammatory stimulation by the dying cell.

The molecular process of apoptosis is energetically costly and is driven by members of the caspase family of proteolytic enzymes (see Section 3.4.4 and Fig. 3.9). In the context of apoptosis, two groups of caspases are crucial, the initiator caspases (e.g., caspase-8 and -9) and the executioner caspases (e.g., caspase-3 and -7). Caspases are also involved in pyroptotic and necroptotic cell death (see Sections 3.5.3 and 3.5.4). Depending on the source of the stimulus, apoptotic cell death can be activated by one of two distinct pathways—the intrinsic or extrinsic pathway (Fig. 3.9). These are sometimes also referred to as the mitochondrial and death-receptor apoptotic pathways, respectively. Although many elements of the two pathways are independent of one another, they are not entirely separate and converge on the final execution stages of the pathway.

The intrinsic apoptotic pathway: The intrinsic pathway can be activated by a vast range of mechanisms and unlike the extrinsic pathway, see below, does not use classic ligand:receptor–based signaling. Activation can result from both positive and negative stimuli, represented by the presence of proapoptotic and the absence of antiapoptotic stimuli respectively. Negative stimuli can include the absence of growth factors and failure to suppress death signaling pathways. Positive stimuli may result from viral infection, cell damage and stress, free radical formation, or ionic changes. Switching on the intrinsic pathway is directly connected to the health and function of the mitochondria as all these stimuli lead to changes in mitochondrial integrity and membrane permeability. The net result of this is the release of proapoptotic molecules in the cytoplasm. This is beautifully exemplified by the release of cytochrome c, which then binds Apaf-1 and causes the protein to form a heptameric wheel-like complex known as the apoptosome that recruits and leads to the activation of pro-caspase-9 (Figs. 3.9 and 3.10). Caspase-9 then activates the executioner caspases, caspase-3, -6, and -7, leading to the terminal degradation of the cell. Other proteins that are released from the mitochondria, such as CAD and endonuclease G, migrate to the nucleus where they induce DNA fragmentation and chromatin condensation.

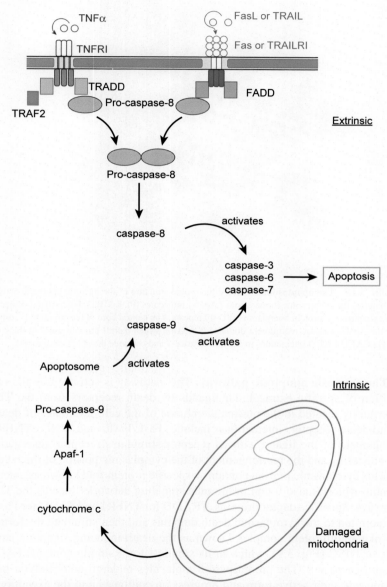

FIGURE 3.9   A simplified overview of the intrinsic and extrinsic apoptotic cell death pathways. Damage to the mitochondria can result in activation of the intrinsic pathway of apoptosis. Apaf-1 recognizes cytochrome c released from the mitochondria, forms a heptameric complex, and recruits pro-caspase-9 to form an apoptosome, which results in caspase-9 activation. Caspase-9 subsequently activates the executioner caspases 3, 6, and 7. In the extrinsic pathway, death receptors in the plasma membrane respond to their ligands to assemble mutliprotein complexes that ultimately result in the activation of caspase-8, which then activates caspase-3, -6, and -7.

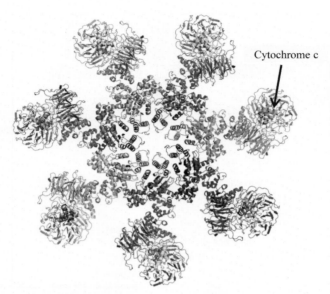

Cytochrome c

FIGURE 3.10 **The apoptosome.** Three-dimensional structure of the intrinsic apoptotic activating complex, the apoptosome formed from 7 Apaf-1 molecules (PDB 3JBT). Each Apaf-1 molecule has a cytochrome c protein bound to its WD-40 repeats. The central core of the structure is formed from the Apaf-1 caspase recruitment domains (CARDs), which recruit pro-caspase-9 to the complex via CARD:CARD interactions to activate caspase-9 and continue the apoptotic cascade.

The extrinsic apoptotic pathway: This pathway is activated by the recognition of specific extracellular ligands by death receptors from the TNF superfamily located in the plasma membrane of the cell. Examples of death-ligand:death-receptor interactions include FasL/FasR and TNFα/TNFR1. Engagement of the ligand with its receptor stimulates receptor aggregation and clustering and the rearrangement of the cytoplasmic portion of the receptor. This cytoplasmic portion contains a specific protein fold known as a death domain, which is also found in immune signaling networks such as the TLR pathways. Specific adaptor proteins, TRADD for TNFR1 and FADD for FasR, are recruited to the cytoplasmic death domains and then stimulate the formation of a multiprotein complex known as the death-inducing signaling complex, or DISC (Fig. 3.9), which in its simplest form simply contains FADD and pro-caspase-8. The pro-caspase-8 molecules undergo autocatalytic processing into their active form and progression continues into the executioner stage of apoptosis via processing of the zymogen forms on the executioner caspases into their active forms.

Regulation and control of apoptosis: Given its fatal nature, it is essential that a cell can regulate and control progression into apoptosis. The intrinsic pathway is heavily controlled by members of the Bcl-2, Bcl-2-like, and IAP families of proteins, and the extrinsic pathway is regulated by the activity of cFLIP, which interferes with DISC assembly and pro-caspase-8 activation. The Bcl-2 and Bcl-2–like families contain a mix of antiapoptotic proteins such as Bcl-2 and proapoptotic proteins such as Bax and Bak. There is also a group of proteins (Bad, Bim, Puma, and Noxa) that form a BH3-only subfamily. These proteins form homo- and heterodimers with one another and work to regulate mitochondrial homeostasis and permeability. Exposure of the cell to stress conditions such as DNA damage, or growth factor and nutrient deprivation, results in the BH3-only proteins interacting with and inactivating the antiapoptotic proteins. This then frees Bak and Bax to enhance membrane permeability to facilitate the release of cytochrome c. The IAP family work by inhibiting caspase activation and by binding and sequestering some of the molecules released from damaged mitochondria. This helps to create a threshold of activation and ensures that apoptosis is not inadvertently activated or taken through to completion unless the level of damage to the cell, or the scale of apoptotic stimulation, is sufficient to overcome these controls.

3.5.2 Necrosis

In stark contrast to apoptosis the process of necrosis is uncontrolled and extremely damaging to the surrounding tissues of the host. In extreme cases, necrotic death can be so severe, and the level of tissue destruction so great, that it can result in death of the host, or situations where the only viable treatment option is amputation of the affected limb. The potentially severe effects of necrosis are readily seen in gangrene. Gangrene often results from injury or infection in which loss of blood circulation to the affected area, often peripheral regions such as toes and fingers, leads to necrotic cell death. It is also increasingly seen in chronic conditions such as atherosclerosis or diabetes, which affect circulatory function. One of the most dramatic manifestations of necrosis occurs with necrotizing fasciitis following infection with certain strains of *Staphylococcus* and *Streptococcus*. Toxins secreted by the bacteria cause rapid death of the surrounding tissues and if not quickly treated may well lead to the induction of sepsis and death.

Necrotic death can be broadly described as the rupture of a cell and the release of its intracellular contents into the surrounding environment. It is often characterized by cell and organelle swelling followed by extensive permeabilization, or rupture, of the plasma membrane. Triggers of necrotic death may include extreme physical or chemical stress such as results from physical trauma, extremes of temperature, large changes in osmotic potential, or be the result of cytolytic toxins. Although one cannot define specific cellular pathways that induce necrosis, it is often observed that intracellular calcium mobilization is heavily disrupted. This is often the result of the cellular stresses inducing mitochondrial calcium overload, which contributes along with various other processes, to mitochondrial dysfunction, the loss of ionic potential, and subsequent failure of the integrity of the plasma membrane. All of these changes lead to a situation in which the cell is unable to control the death process and therefore necrosis leads to the release of a large range of potentially harmful lytic enzymes, proteases, free radicals, and reactive oxygen and nitrogen species, which can themselves be directly damaging to the surrounding tissues. Necrotic death also releases DAMPs, which will then be detected by PRRs and lead to the activation of proinflammatory signaling pathways and the recruitment of inflammatory cells such as macrophages and neutrophils to the site of damage. This can lead to resolution and repair of the damage associated with necrosis, but may also serve to exacerbate the damage caused.

3.5.3 Necroptosis

The term necroptosis is used to describe the process of controlled necrosis and therefore appears to be somewhat of a physiological contradiction. Microscopically, cells undergoing necroptosis are indistinguishable from those dying as a result of necrosis. Both populations display swollen organelles and swollen cells, which lead to membrane permeabilization and rupture. Given the broadly harmful effects of necrosis summarized in Section 3.5.2, it seems counterintuitive that the host would ever want to deliberately initiate such a potentially damaging manner of cell death. However, it is clear that the induction of necroptosis is actually a surprisingly common pathway employed by cells in response to a range of threat and danger-related stimuli. For example, signaling via the cell surface IFN-receptor and TNF-receptor, the intracellular PRR TLR3 and the cytoplasmic PRR DAI have all been shown to be capable of inducing necroptosis. The widespread expression of these receptors implies that necroptosis should occur with a high frequency. However, under most circumstances the progression to necroptosis stalls because of the tight control of the downstream signaling processes. This control is mediated by a number of intracellular proteins, which includes caspase-8, c-FLIP$_L$, cIAP1, and cIAP2. Consequently, necroptotic death will only occur if the regulatory activities of these proteins are blocked. Cells are, in essence, primed to enter necroptosis but unable to progress until the appropriate permissions are given. This can happen following the further activation of PRR signaling pathways or directly as a result of the action of pathogen-derived proteins.

Our understanding of the molecular and structural basis of necroptosis has been rapidly improving over recent years. The general necroptotic pathway is illustrated in Fig. 3.11. One of the key proteins involved in the induction of necroptosis, particularly via TNF-dependant pathways, is the serine/threonine kinase RIPK1. Activation of RIPK1 leads to the subsequent activation of RIPK3 and the formation of a macromolecular complex known as the ripoptosome. The late events in necroptosis appear to be heavily dependent on the protein mixed-lineage kinase domain-like protein (MLKL), which has been described as an effector molecule for necroptosis. Once RIPK3 has been activated, it phosphorylates MLKL, which leads to MLKL oligomerization and the subsequent permeabilization of the membrane.

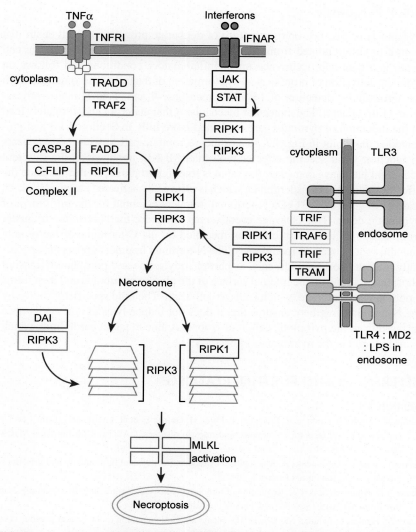

FIGURE 3.11   The necroptotic cell death pathway. The formation of a necrosome from RIPK1 and RIPK3 is the key event in initiating necroptosis as this structure serves to activate mixed-lineage kinase domain-like protein (MLKL), which then perturbs the cell membrane to induce death. Necrosome formation can be induced by some intracellular nucleic acid sensors such as DAI; through toll/interleukin-1 resistance domain–containing adaptor inducing interferon β (TRIF)-dependent pathways from TLR3 or TLR4 at the endosomal membrane; as a result of IFN signaling; and through the activation of death receptors.

3.5.4 Pyroptosis

Pyroptosis is, like necroptosis, a form of deliberate programmed cell death that cannot be differentiated from necrosis at the microscopic level. Pyroptotic cell death is a common occurrence under inflammatory conditions and follows on from the activation of procaspase-1 via formation of the inflammasome, and from the intracellular detection of LPS by procaspase-4 and -5 in humans (procaspase-11 in rodents). The molecular mechanisms that underpin and ultimately lead to the induction of pyroptosis are explained more fully in Section 4.1.3 and presented at that point in Fig. 4.7. Just as the necroptotic pathway currently appears to function via a specific effector molecule, MLKL, upon which the different activation pathways converge, the same is true in pyroptosis. In this instance the effector molecule is Gasdermin D, which is cleaved by activated caspase-1, -4, -5, and -11 to generate a 31 kDa N-terminal fragment essential for the fulfillment of pyroptotic death. This cleavage event serves to release the N-terminal fragment from an autoinhibited conformation mediated by the C-terminus of the protein and allows it relocate to membranes. The N-terminal fragment appears to specifically bind to phospholipids, such as phosphatidylserine and phosphatidylinositol phosphates, found on the internal surface of the plasma membrane and then forms a pore in the membrane, which leads to cell death. The lipid specificity shown by the N-terminal fragment ensures that it does not induce lysis in other cells once released from the pyroptotic cell. It also appears able to target cardiolipin, which is often found in the membranes of bacteria.

REFERENCES AND FURTHER READING

Section 3.1

Akdis M, Burgler S, Crameri R, Eiwegger T, Fujita H, Gomez E, et al. Interleukins, from 1 to 37, and interferon-γ: receptors, functions, and roles in diseases. J Allergy Clin Immunol March 2011;127(3):701–21.e70.

Arango Duque G, Descoteaux A. Macrophage cytokines: involvement in immunity and infectious diseases. Front Immunol October 7, 2014;5.

Brenner D, Blaser H, Mak TW. Regulation of tumour necrosis factor signalling: live or let die. Nat Rev Immunol 2015;15(6):362–74. Nature Publishing Group.

Carty M, Reinert L, Paludan SR, Bowie AG. Innate antiviral signalling in the central nervous system. Trends Immunol February 2014;35(2):79–87.

Chow KT, Gale M. SnapShot: interferon signaling. Cell December 2015;163(7):1808–1808.e1.

Clore GM, Appella E, Yamada M, Matsushima K, Gronenborn AM. Three-dimensional structure of interleukin 8 in solution. Biochemistry February 20, 1990;29(7):1689–96.

Eck MJ, Sprang SR. The structure of tumor necrosis factor-alpha at 2.6 A resolution. Implications for receptor binding. J Biol Chem October 15, 1989;264(29):17595–605.

Finzel BC, Clancy LL, Holland DR, Muchmore SW, Watenpaugh KD, Einspahr HM. Crystal structure of recombinant human interleukin-1 beta at 2.0 A resolution. J Mol Biol October 20, 1989;209(4):779–91.

Garlanda C, Dinarello CA, Mantovani A. The interleukin-1 family: back to the future. Immunity December 2013;39(6):1003–18.

Hand TW. Interleukin-18: the bouncer at the mucosal bar. Cell December 2015;163(6):1310–2.

Ivashkiv LB, Donlin LT. Regulation of type I interferon responses. Nat Rev Immunol December 23, 2013;14(1):36–49.

Jurk M, Heil F, Vollmer J, Schetter C, Krieg AM, Wagner H, et al. Human TLR7 or TLR8 independently confer responsiveness to the antiviral compound R-848. Nat Immunol 2002;3(6):499.

Kraich M, Klein M, Patiño E, Harrer H, Nickel J, Sebald W, et al. A modular interface of IL-4 allows for scalable affinity without affecting specificity for the IL-4 receptor. BMC Biol 2006;4:13.

Lafyatis R. Transforming growth factor β—at the centre of systemic sclerosis. Nat Rev Rheumatol August 19, 2014;10(12):706–19.

LaPorte SL, Juo ZS, Vaclavikova J, Colf LA, Qi X, Heller NM, et al. Molecular and structural basis of cytokine receptor pleiotropy in the interleukin-4/13 system. Cell January 25, 2008;132(2):259–72.

Liu S, Song X, Chrunyk BA, Shanker S, Hoth LR, Marr ES, et al. Crystal structures of interleukin 17A and its complex with IL-17 receptor A. Nat Commun 2013;4:1888.

Menten P, Wuyts A, Van Damme J. Macrophage inflammatory protein-1. Cytokine Growth Factor Rev December 2002;13(6):455–81.

Mukai Y, Nakamura T, Yoshikawa M, Yoshioka Y, Tsunoda S, Nakagawa S, et al. Solution of the structure of the TNF-TNFR2 complex. Sci Signal 2010;3(148):ra83.

Nilsberth C, Elander L, Hamzic N, Norell M, Lönn J, Engström L, et al. The role of interleukin-6 in lipopolysaccharide-induced fever by mechanisms independent of prostaglandin E2. Endocrinology April 2009;150(4):1850–60.

Palomo J, Dietrich D, Martin P, Palmer G, Gabay C. The interleukin (IL)-1 cytokine family – balance between agonists and antagonists in inflammatory diseases. Cytokine 2015;76(1):25–37. Elsevier Ltd.

Randal M, Kossiakoff AA. The 2.0 A structure of bovine interferon-gamma; assessment of the structural differences between species. Acta Crystallogr D Biol Crystallogr January 2000;56(Pt 1):14–24.

Redpath SA, Heieis G, Perona-Wright G. Spatial regulation of IL-4 signalling in vivo. Cytokine September 2015;75(1):51–6.

Schoggins JW, Wilson SJ, Panis M, Murphy MY, Jones CT, Bieniasz P, et al. A diverse range of gene products are effectors of the type I interferon antiviral response. Nature April 28, 2011;472(7344):481–5. Nature Publishing Group, A Division of Macmillan Publishers Limited. All Rights Reserved.

Šedý J, Bekiaris V, Ware CF. Tumor necrosis factor superfamily in innate immunity and inflammation. Cold Spring Harb Perspect Biol April 2015;7(4):a016279.

Sokol CL, Luster AD. The chemokine system in innate immunity. Cold Spring Harb Perspect Biol May 2015;7(5):a016303.

Thomas C, Bazan JF, Garcia KC. Structure of the activating IL-1 receptor signaling complex. Nat Struct Mol Biol April 2012;19(4):455–7.

Thomas C, Moraga I, Levin D, Krutzik PO, Podoplelova Y, Trejo A, et al. Structural linkage between ligand discrimination and receptor activation by type I interferons. Cell August 2011;146(4):621–32.

Tsutsumi N, Kimura T, Arita K, Ariyoshi M, Ohnishi H, Yamamoto T, et al. The structural basis for receptor recognition of human interleukin-18. Nat Commun 2014;5:5340.

Turner MD, Nedjai B, Hurst T, Pennington DJ. Cytokines and chemokines: at the crossroads of cell signalling and inflammatory disease. Biochim Biophys Acta November 2014;1843(11):2563–82.

Van Dyken SJ, Locksley RM. Interleukin-4- and interleukin-13-mediated alternatively activated macrophages: roles in homeostasis and disease. Annu Rev Immunol March 21, 2013;31(1):317–43.

Walter MR. The molecular basis of IL-10 function: from receptor structure to the onset of signaling. Curr Top Microbiol Immunol 2014:191–212.

Ward-Kavanagh LK, Lin WW, Šedý JR, Ware CF. The TNF receptor superfamily in co-stimulating and co-inhibitory responses. Immunity May 2016;44(5):1005–19.

Wicks IP, Roberts AW. Targeting GM-CSF in inflammatory diseases. Nat Rev Rheumatol December 3, 2015;12(1):37–48.

Yao Y, Tsirka SE. Monocyte chemoattractant protein-1 and the blood–brain barrier. Cell Mol Life Sci February 20, 2014;71(4):683–97.

Sections 3.2–3.5

Aglietti RA, Estevez A, Gupta A, Ramirez MG, Liu PS, Kayagaki N, et al. GsdmD p30 elicited by caspase-11 during pyroptosis forms pores in membranes. Proc Natl Acad Sci USA June 23, 2016;113(28):7858–63.

Ashkenazi A, Salvesen G. Regulated cell death: signaling and mechanisms. Annu Rev Cell Dev Biol 2014;30:337–56.

Bajic G, Degn SE, Thiel S, Andersen GR. Complement activation, regulation, and molecular basis for complement-related diseases. EMBO J 2015;34(22):1–23.

Bryan N, Ahswin H, Smart N, Bayon Y, Wohlert S, Hunt JA. Reactive oxygen species (ROS)–a family of fate deciding molecules pivotal in constructive inflammation and wound healing. Eur Cell Mater 2012;24:249–65.

Cray C. Acute phase proteins in animals. Prog Mol Biol Transl Sci 2012;105:113–50.

Dennis EA, Norris PC. Eicosanoid storm in infection and inflammation. Nat Rev Immunol 2015;15(8):511–23. Nature Publishing Group.

Ding J, Wang K, Liu W, She Y, Sun Q, Shi J, et al. Pore-forming activity and structural autoinhibition of the gasdermin family. Nature June 8, 2016;535(7610):111–6.

Elmore S. Apoptosis: a review of programmed cell death. Toxicol Pathol June 2007;35(4):495–516.

Engelmann B, Massberg S. Thrombosis as an intravascular effector of innate immunity. Nat Rev Immunol January 2013;13(1):34–45.

Fuchs Y, Steller H. Live to die another way: modes of programmed cell death and the signals emanating from dying cells. Nat Rev Mol Cell Biol 2015;16(6):329–44. Nature Publishing Group.

Fuchs Y, Steller H. Programmed cell death in animal development and disease. Cell November 2011;147(4):742–58.

Gabay C, Kushner I. Acute-phase proteins and other systemic responses to inflammation. N Engl J Med February 11, 1999;340(6):448–54.

Goldar S, Khaniani MS, Derakhshan SM, Baradaran B. Molecular mechanisms of apoptosis and roles in cancer development and treatment. Asian Pac J Cancer Prev April 3, 2015;16(6):2129–44.

Harijith A, Ebenezer DL, Natarajan V. Reactive oxygen species at the crossroads of inflammasome and inflammation. Front Physiol 2014;5:352.

Iwanaga S, Kawabata S. Evolution and phylogeny of defense molecules associated with innate immunity in horseshoe crab. Front Biosci September 1, 1998;3:D973–84.

Liu X, Zhang Z, Ruan J, Pan Y, Magupalli VG, Wu H, et al. Inflammasome-activated gasdermin D causes pyroptosis by forming membrane pores. Nature July 7, 2016;535(7610):153–8.

Lu J, Yu Y, Zhu I, Cheng Y, Sun PD. Structural mechanism of serum amyloid A-mediated inflammatory amyloidosis. Proc Natl Acad Sci USA April 8, 2014;111(14):5189–94.

Merle NS, Church SE, Fremeaux-Bacchi V, Roumenina LT. Complement system part I – molecular mechanisms of activation and regulation. Front Immunol 2015;6:262.

Merle NS, Noe R, Halbwachs-Mecarelli L, Fremeaux-Bacchi V, Roumenina LT. Complement system part II: role in immunity. Front Immunol 2015;6:257.

Shrive AK, Cheetham GM, Holden D, Myles DA, Turnell WG, Volanakis JE, et al. Three dimensional structure of human C-reactive protein. Nat Struct Biol April 1996;3(4):346–54.

Silke J, Rickard JA, Gerlic M. The diverse role of RIP kinases in necroptosis and inflammation. Nat Immunol June 18, 2015;16(7):689–97.

van der Poll T, Herwald H. The coagulation system and its function in early immune defense. Thromb Haemost October 2014;112(4):640–8.

Versteeg HH, Heemskerk JWM, Levi M, Reitsma PH. New fundamentals in hemostasis. Physiol Rev January 1, 2013;93(1):327–58.

Wallach D, Kang T-B, Dillon CP, Green DR. Programmed necrosis in inflammation: toward identification of the effector molecules. Science April 1, 2016;352(6281):aaf2154.

Witkowski M, Landmesser U, Rauch U. Tissue factor as a link between inflammation and coagulation. Trends Cardiovasc Med May 2016;26(4):297–303.

Zhou M, Li Y, Hu Q, Bai X-C, Huang W, Yan C, et al. Atomic structure of the apoptosome: mechanism of cytochrome c- and dATP-mediated activation of Apaf-1. Genes Dev November 15, 2015;29(22):2349–61.

Section 4

Integrated Innate Immunity— Combining Activation and Effector Functions

4.1 THE DETECTION OF BACTERIAL LIPOPOLYSACCHARIDE

LPS is one of the most potent immune stimuli known. It is found in the outer membrane of Gram-negative bacteria, such as *Escherichia coli, Salmonella* spp., *Vibrio cholera*, and *Neisseria* spp., where it provides critical structural and functional roles. It is the major cause of septic shock resulting from systemic Gram-negative bacterial infection. LPS is composed of three distinct domains: a membrane anchored lipid A portion, a central polysaccharide core, and a distal O-antigen, or O-polysaccharide, component (Fig. 4.1). Each of these regions has a distinct functional role to play, and both the lipid A and O-antigen regions interface with the immune system.

Biochemically the lipid A portion of LPS consists of a phosphorylated diglucosamine backbone to which acyl chains are attached (Fig. 4.1). The acyl chains confer the hydrophobic properties of lipid A that allow it to insert and anchor in the outer bacterial membrane. Up to four acyl chains can be attached directly to the diglucosamine sugar by means of either an ester or amide linkage. These acyl chains are almost always saturated and may include substitutions that include the attachment of additional acyl chains. *E. coli*, for example, has a total of four acyl chains extending from one sugar and two from the other, whereas *Neisseria meningitidis* has three chains extending from each. Lipid A is commonly referred to as endotoxin and it is this component that functions as a voracious activator of the innate immune system. The exact immunogenicity of the lipid A component is determined by the precise nature and number of the substitutions on the acyl chains. For example, hexaacylated *E. coli* LPS is strongly immunogenic (Fig. 4.1B), whereas LPS from *Helicobacter pylori* is not. The reduced immunogenicity of *H. pylori* LPS is the result of substitutions of the phosphate groups, longer acyl chains, and the presence of forms with only four, or indeed only one, acyl chain.

The terms LPS, lipid A, and endotoxin, are routinely used in an interchangeable manner within the field of immunology. It has long been known that extracellular LPS triggers proinflammatory signaling via activation of the pattern

The Innate Immune System. http://dx.doi.org/10.1016/B978-0-12-804464-3.00004-1

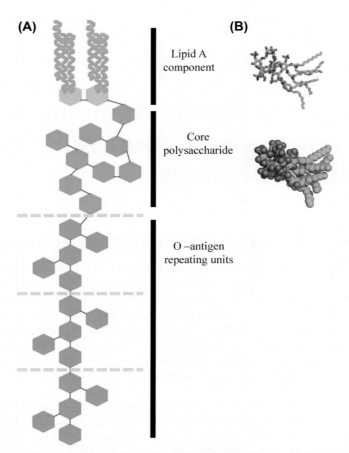

FIGURE 4.1   The organization of lipopolysaccharide (LPS) from Gram-negative bacteria. (A) LPS consists of a lipid A component (orange) containing a core disaccharide with attached acyl groups. The number and type of acyl chains show some variation between bacterial strains. This is the immunogenic portion of LPS and is often referred to as endotoxin. It is usually inserted into the outer membrane of Gram-negative bacteria. Lipid A is attached to a core region of polysaccharides (green), which is in turn anchored to an outer region of repeating polysaccharide units known as the O-antigen or O-polysaccharide (purple). The O-antigen is highly variable in composition. (B) Structures of the lipid A portion of *Escherichia coli* LPS shown in *stick* (top panel) and *sphere* (lower panel) representations. The acyl chains extend to the right of the molecule. Structural details are derived from the PDB file 3FXI and carbon atoms are cyan, oxygen atoms are red, phosphorous atoms are orange, nitrogen atoms are blue, and hydrogens are not shown. Monosaccharides are represented as hexagons.

recognition receptor (PRR) TLR4. However, it has only recently come to light that LPS that becomes intracellular also triggers an innate immune response following its detection by members of the inflammatory caspases, specifically, caspase-11 in rodents and caspase-4 and -5 in primates. Excessive activation of these pathways can lead to sepsis, and endotoxin is generally accepted to be the major driver of Gram-negative bacteria–associated septic shock.

Lipid A is connected to the core polysaccharide region of LPS. This linkage is invariably mediated by between one and three KDO residues (an 8 carbon ketose—2-keto-3-deoxy-octanoic acid). The linkage bonds are relatively acid labile and therefore break readily to release the lipid A portion when the LPS molecule dissociates, or is released from, the bacterial membrane. The composition of the core polysaccharide region shows a high level of conservation between different species and strains of bacteria. The KDO residues adjacent to lipid A are often accompanied by heptose sugars and together form the inner core region. The outer core, which is adjacent to the O-antigen component (Fig. 4.1), is commonly found to consist of sugars such as galactose, glucose, and N-acetylated versions of glucosamine and galactosamine.

The part of LPS most distal from the bacterial membrane is the O-antigen region. This consists of a variable number of repeating subunits formed from between one to eight monosaccharides (Fig. 4.1). The type, number, and linkage of these monosaccharides show extremely high levels of variation and therefore result in the O-antigen displaying widely heterogeneous immunological characteristics. Given that the O-antigen is the major target for antibodies against LPS, this variability serves as an immune evasion mechanism for the bacteria and helps to neutralize the efficiency of LPS-targeting antibodies generated by the adaptive immune response.

4.1.1 Activation of TLR4 Signaling by Extracellular Lipopolysaccharide

When anchored within the outer membrane of Gram-negative bacteria, the lipid A portion of LPS is not accessible for immune recognition by either acute phase proteins or pattern recognition receptors. However, LPS can be shed from bacteria as they grow and replicate, when they release outer membrane vesicles, or when they die. At this point the lipid A portion is commonly released from the bacterial membrane and becomes a viable target for immune recognition.

Activation of TLR4 signaling by LPS is a multiprotein process and is summarized in Fig. 4.2. The structures of the major players in this process are provided in Fig. 4.3. Once free in the serum, LPS is bound by the acute phase protein LPS-binding protein (LBP), which, like many acute phase proteins is synthesized in the liver (Figs. 4.2 and 4.3). LBP is a glycosylated protein of approximately 60 kDa. It has two primary functions. One of these is to limit inflammation by transferring LPS to lipoproteins that serve to neutralize the inflammatory potential of the molecule, most likely by masking the lipid A component. The second role is to promote inflammation by facilitating the recognition of LPS by the leucine-rich repeat containing protein CD14 (Figs. 4.2 and 4.3). CD14 exists as a membrane-anchored protein on the surface of cells, particularly immune cells, but also occurs in a soluble form free in the serum (Fig. 4.2). CD14 acts to greatly enhance the affinity with which LPS can bind to the MD-2:TLR4 complex. The precise mechanism by which this enhancement occurs remains unclear, but in the absence of CD14, mice are protected against LPS-induced septic shock. It is most likely that CD14 serves to catalyze the

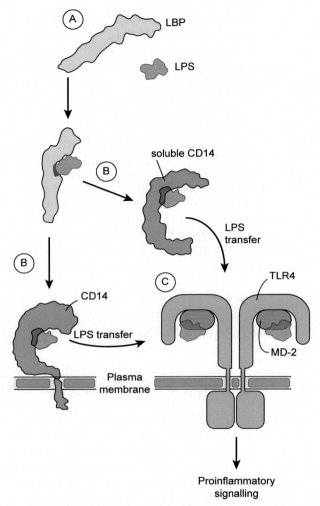

FIGURE 4.2 Schematic illustration of the recognition of extracellular lipopolysaccharide (LPS). The lipid A component of bacterial LPS in the serum is bound in a C-terminal groove of the LPS-binding protein, LBP (A) and then transferred to CD14 (B), which can be presented in a soluble form free in solution or as a membrane-bound form. LPS is then transferred to the hydrophobic pocket of MD-2, which is in complex with the extracellular leucine-rich repeat–containing ectodomain of TLR4 (C). The final signaling competent complex forms an M shape and contains two copies of each of the TLR4, MD-2, and LPS molecules. This causes activation of the Toll-like receptor signaling pathway and production of proinflammatory cytokines. LPS can be recruited to MD-2 independently of LBP and also CD14; however, in the presence of CD14 the process is much more efficient and the resulting signaling cascade, more effective.

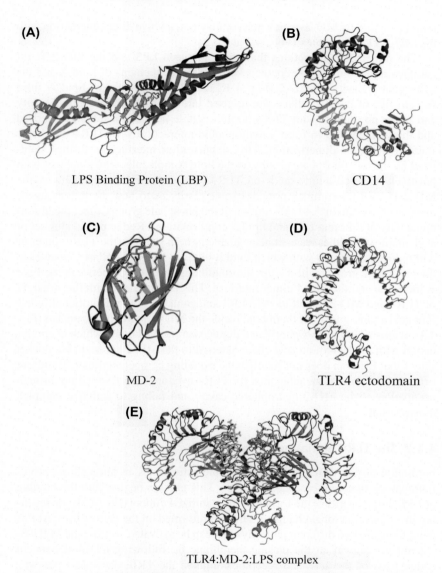

FIGURE 4.3 **The structural basis of extracellular lipopolysaccharide (LPS) detection.** Cartoon representations of the three-dimensional structures of the key proteins involved in the detection of extracellular LPS. (A) Murine LBP with lipid bound in a C-terminal hydrophobic groove. (B) The ligand-free conformation of the murine CD14 leucine-rich repeats. (C) Human MD-2 with lipid-IVa bound in the hydrophobic pocket. (D) The extracellular ectodomain of human TLR4. (E) The active M-shaped form of the MD-2:TLR4:LPS complex. In each image, alpha helices are colored raspberry red, beta sheets are slate blue, and loop regions are gray. The ligands bound in panels A, C, and E are colored orange and presented as stick representations. The PDB files used are (A) murine LBP—4M4D; (B) murine CD14—1WWL; (C) human MD-2 and lipid IVa—2E59; (D) human TLR4 ectodomain—3FXI; (E) TLR4:MD-2:LPS complex—3FXI.

binding of LPS by MD-2, which may, or may not, involve direct interaction with the MD-2:TLR4 complex (Figs. 4.2 and 4.3).

The molecular interactions that occur between LPS and the MD-2:TLR4 complex are dominated by contacts between the acyl chains of lipid A and the hydrophobic cavity of MD-2 (Fig. 4.3C and E). In the case of lipid A from *E. coli*, five of the acyl chains are inserted into the MD-2 hydrophobic cavity and make no contact with TLR4. Only a single acyl chain remains exposed and this is then able to form a hydrophobic interaction with TLR4 that helps stabilize receptor dimerization. This dimerization interface is further stabilized by the two phosphate groups on the lipid A molecule, which interact with positively charged amino acids on TLR4. The structural arrangement of the MD-2:TLR4:LPS complex provides some clarity as to how alterations in the number of acyl chains and substitution of the phosphate groups affect the immunogenicity of different LPS and lipid A conformations. Reducing the number of acyl chains will either leave none available to help stabilize the TLR4 dimer or will reduce the affinity with which lipid A binds to MD-2. Similarly, changes to the phosphate groups will disrupt the stabilizing interactions between the lipid A molecule and the TLR4 dimer interface. This is consistent with the structure of TLR4 and MD-2 bound to the TLR4 antagonist Eritoran. Eritoran only has four acyl chains and all of them bind inside the MD-2 hydrophobic pocket (Fig. 4.4). It also lacks the phosphorylated diglucosamine backbone, which in combination with the lack of an acyl chain external to the MD-2 hydrophobic pocket shows that Eritoran does not stabilize the signaling competent dimer. Therefore Eritoran functions as an antagonist for TLR4 by stopping LPS binding through occupation of the MD-2 hydrophobic cavity and failing to stabilize complex dimerization.

4.1.2 The TLR4 Signaling Pathway

Formation of the MD-2:TLR4:LPS complex stimulates an intracellular proinflammatory signaling cascade (Fig. 4.5). This process begins with the binding of LPS inducing either the formation of stabilized dimers (Fig. 4.3E) or resulting in a conformational change in dimers preformed on the cell surface. At this point there are two different pathways that can be activated—either the MyD88-dependent pathway at the plasma membrane or, following CD14–dependent endocytosis of the activated receptor complex, the TRIF-dependent pathway from the endosomal membrane (Fig. 4.5).

The dimeric MD-2:TLR4:LPS complexes have a characteristic "m"-shape, and it is likely that this arrangement is required to allow adoption of the correct conformation of the transmembrane helices and the intracellular Toll/interleukin-1 resistance (TIR) domains to permit downstream signaling. The TIR domains of each TLR4 molecule most likely interact to form a dimer that can then act as a platform for the recruitment of the necessary additional proteins required for signaling. The precise spatial conformation

(A)

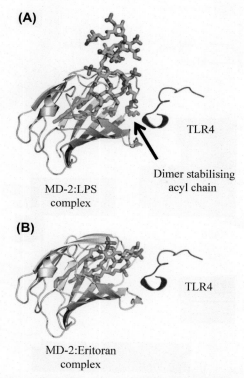

TLR4

Dimer stabilising
acyl chain

MD-2:LPS
complex

(B)

TLR4

MD-2:Eritoran
complex

FIGURE 4.4 **Eritoran is an antagonist of lipopolysaccharide (LPS)-driven TLR4 activation.** (A) The complex of MD-2 and LPS has five acyl chains in the MD-2 hydrophobic pocket and one (marked by an arrow) outside the pocket and able to make stabilizing contacts with part of TLR4. (B) When Eritoran binds to MD-2, all four of its acyl chains are inside the hydrophobic pocket and cannot help stabilize the formation of the TLR4 signaling complex. Images generated from PDBs 3FXI (MD-2:LPS) and 2Z65 (MD-2:Eritoran).

of the TLR4 TIR domains remains uncertain, but dimeric structures have been solved for the TIRs of TLR6 and TLR10 (Fig. 4.6) and therefore provide insight into the potential conformations that might be adopted. What is clear is that a region of the TLR4 TIR known as the BB loop is absolutely crucial for the propagation of signal transduction. Mutations in this region result in a loss of signaling. This is clearly demonstrated by the fact that the identity of TLR4 as a receptor for LPS was first recognized based on the inability of mice containing a P714H mutation in the BB loop of the TLR4 TIR to respond to LPS.

Following activation, TLR4 follows two signaling pathways—one from the plasma membrane and the other from the endosomal membrane after internalization of the receptor complex (Fig. 4.5). Signaling at the plasma membrane involves recruitment of the bridging adaptor Mal to the TIR

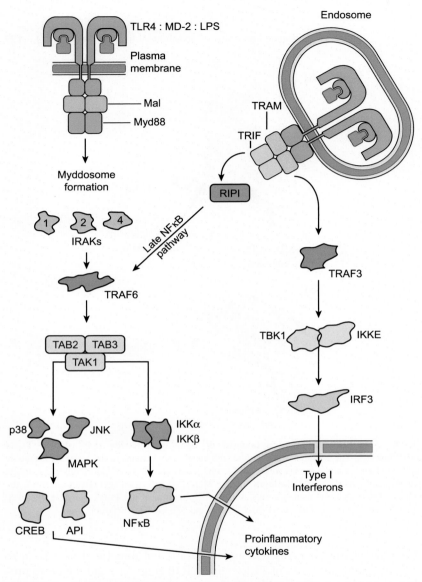

FIGURE 4.5 A schematic illustration of the TLR4 signaling pathway. Activation of the MD-2:TLR4:LPS complex takes place at the plasma membrane. This can lead either to signal transduction initiated from the plasma membrane (A), or the endocytosis of the MD-2:TLR4:LPS complex and subsequent signaling from the endosomal membrane (B). Signaling from the plasma membrane requires recruitment of the bridging adaptor Mal to the TLR4 Toll/interleukin-1 resistance domains, which then recruit MyD88. MyD88 interacts with IRAK4, IRAK1, and IRAK2 to form the Myddosome complex. Signaling continues via the involvement of TNF receptor–associated factors (TRAFs), TGFβ-activated kinase 1 (TAK1), and TAK1-binding proteins (TABs). This ultimately activates stress kinase and NFκB signaling pathways to stimulate proinflammatory gene expression. Signaling from the endosomal membrane involves the recruitment of two different adaptor proteins, TRAM and TRIF, and signals via TRAF3 to activate the IRF3 transcription factor and stimulate the production of type I IFNs. Endosomal TLR4 can also activate the stress kinase and NFκB pathways by recruiting receptor-interacting protein 1 to the TRAM and TRIF adaptors. This pathway results in delayed proinflammatory gene expression when compared to signaling from the plasma membrane.

(A)   **(B)**

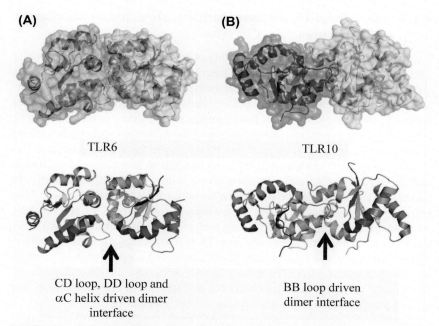

TLR6   TLR10

CD loop, DD loop and   BB loop driven
αC helix driven dimer   dimer interface
interface

FIGURE 4.6   TLR TIR domains can form dimeric structures that may function as molecular scaffolds for downstream signaling. The TLR6 (A) and TLR10 (B) TIR domain structures have been solved using X-ray crystallography. In both cases the structures revealed a dimeric complex; however, their interaction surfaces differ. The dimer interface in the TLR6 structure is formed from contacts between the CD loop, DD loop, and alphaC helix from both monomers. In contrast, the TLR10 dimer interface is dominated by interaction between the BB loops. Each structure is presented as a cartoon and surface representation (top panels) and a cartoon representation only (bottom panel). Each monomer in the bottom panel is colored blue to red from the N-terminus of the protein to further highlight the different structural elements in the dimer interface. The TLR6 images are generated from PDB 4OM7 and the TLR10 images from PDB 2J67.

dimer, which in turn recruits MyD88, leading to initiation of Myddosome formation and the induction of an early NFκB-driven inflammatory response. Understandably the process of receptor endocytosis creates a delay in the initiation of signal transduction from the endosomal membrane. In contrast to signaling at the plasma membrane, endosomal TLR4 recruits a separate adaptor protein, TRAM, which in turn recruits the protein TRIF and leads to the formation of a multiprotein complex sometimes referred to as the Triffosome. Endosomal TLR4 signaling does ultimately induce proinflammatory cytokines through classical NFκB signaling pathways, albeit in a delayed manner. However, its primary signaling output is IFN-β following activation of the transcription factor IRF3 (Fig. 4.5). A more detailed description of the general Toll-like receptor (TLR) signaling pathways can be found in Section 2.2.4.

4.1.3 Intracellular Lipopolysaccharide Is Detected by Members of the Inflammatory Caspases

It is only in the last few years that the ability of host cells to recognize intracellular LPS in a TLR-independent manner has been confirmed. LPS is able to enter cells via a variety of routes. For example, membrane permeabilization by bacterial toxins, such as cholera toxin B, permits LPS translocation; LPS can be injected via bacterial secretion systems; LPS from bacteria in endosomes or vacuoles can be released into the cytoplasm; and the fusion of bacterial outer membrane vesicles with the plasma membrane can deliver LPS directly to the cytoplasm (Fig. 4.7).

Once inside the cytoplasm, LPS is recognized by the caspase recruitment domain (CARD) of specific members of the inflammatory caspase family. In humans this function can be performed by both caspase-4 and caspase-5. The homologues in rodents and cows are caspase-11 and caspase-13, respectively. As much of the research has so far been performed using murine cells and models, I will predominantly refer to caspase-11. It is likely, however, that the observations with caspase-11 are broadly applicable to homologous proteins in other species. The use of a CARD for the purposes of caspase-11–dependent detection of LPS represents a major functional deviation from the usual role of this type of protein fold in mediating protein:protein interactions.

Binding of LPS by the caspase-11 CARD involves basic positively charged lysine residues and stimulates aggregation of the protein. The molecular basis of this aggregation is not currently known, but given the multiple interaction surfaces available for CARD-mediated interactions, it may well be driven by CARD:CARD interactions. This behavior can be recapitulated using in vitro protein expression systems. Expressing recombinant caspase-11 CARD using *E. coli*, and therefore in the presence of LPS, causes protein aggregation. This does not happen when using LPS-free insect cells.

The aggregation of LPS serves to bring the catalytic domains into close enough proximity that they can stimulate autoprocessing of the caspase-11 molecules, thereby releasing the active protease. The key substrate for caspase-11 appears to be a cytoplasmic protein called Gasdermin D. Cleavage of Gasdermin D by caspase-11 creates an N-terminal fragment 31 kDa in size. This fragment is a key, maybe the key, determinant in the initiation of pyroptotic cell death. Activation of caspase-11 also results in stimulation of the NLRP3 inflammasome and the production of IL-1β and IL-18. Whether this results from pyroptosis-associated membrane permeabilization or some other form of homeostatic disruption remains to be worked out (Fig. 4.7).

4.2 INTERLEUKIN 1β IS PRODUCED FOLLOWING ACTIVATION OF THE INFLAMMASOME

The inflammasome was very briefly introduced in Section 2.2.6.2. To reiterate, this large multiprotein complex forms in the cytoplasm and can reach sizes of up to a micron in diameter. It has a heterogeneous composition and at the

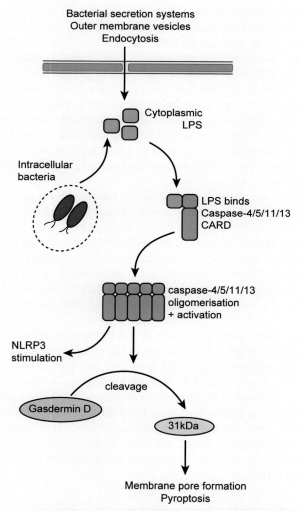

FIGURE 4.7 **The intracellular detection of lipopolysaccharide (LPS) is carried out by members of the inflammatory caspase family.** Bacterial LPS can enter the cytoplasm via various routes including direct bacterial invasion, action of bacterial secretion systems, LPS release from phagocytic or endocytic vesicles, and following membrane fusion with bacterial outer membrane vesicles. Once in the cytoplasm, LPS is recognized by the caspase recruitment domain (CARD) of specific inflammatory caspases—caspase-11 in rodents, caspase-4 and caspase-5 in primates, and caspase-13 in cows. This stimulates caspase aggregation and autoactivation. The active caspase domains are then freed to cleave the cytoplasmic protein Gasdermin D and release a 31-kDa N-terminal fragment that drives cell death by pyroptosis and can contribute to sepsis. The cellular changes induced also activate the NLRP3 inflammasome leading to caspase-1 activation and the production of the proinflammatory cytokines IL-1β and IL-18.

most basic level requires the presence of sensor, adaptor, and effector proteins. Sensors are either specific members of the NLR family or the PYHIN protein AIM2. Of the NLR proteins NLRP1, NLRP3, and NAIP/NLRC4 all definitely trigger inflammasome formation, and it has been suggested that NLRP6, NLRP7, and NLRP12 can also do so, although as yet there is insufficient evidence to conclusively support this. The principal adaptor protein is ASC and in fact inflammasomes are sometimes referred to as ASC specks. However, NLRC4 also functions as an adaptor in the NAIP/NLRC4 inflammasome. Effector proteins take the form of caspases, predominantly caspase-1, although caspase-5 and caspase-8 are known to be recruited to some inflammasomes. The precise composition of the inflammasome is likely to be dynamic, changing over the course of the innate response.

Activation of the inflammasome occurs via a wide range of exogenous and endogenous danger signals. These include classical pathogen-associated molecular patterns (PAMPs) and danger/damage-associated molecular patterns (DAMPs) but also crystalline materials and processes that cause homeostatic disruption (Table 4.1). The assembly of the inflammasome is driven by extensive networks of protein–protein interactions in which the formation of filamentous structures are believed to be a critical element. The overall architecture of the endogenous inflammasome has been shown to be ringlike in nature.

The primary physiological function of the inflammasome is to activate the proteolytic enzyme caspase-1, which in turn can process Gasdermin D (Section 3.5.4) to initiate pyroptosis, and both pro-IL-1β and pro-IL-18 to their active proinflammatory forms (Fig. 4.8). The inflammasome is therefore a critical innate immune response to the presence of danger that produces a proinflammatory response and can lead to cell death. Long-term, or uncontrolled, activation of the inflammasome has been connected with numerous chronic inflammatory conditions (Section 6). Here I will focus on the mechanisms by which the inflammasome can be activated to facilitate the production of the key inflammatory mediator IL-1β.

4.2.1 Activation of the Inflammasome

Inflammasome activation can be brought about by many different exogenous and endogenous stimuli, examples of which are provided in Table 4.1. Scanning the repertoire of activating ligands rapidly reveals that while the NLRP1, NAIP/NLRC4, and AIM2 inflammasomes have very specific ligands, this is not the case for NLRP3. In fact as we shall see the presence, or otherwise, of a specific ligand for NLRP3 remains a contentious issue. Certainly the wide range of ligands and physiological effects known to stimulate NLRP3 inflammasome formation share no basic structural, biological, or chemical similarity. At the moment, it is therefore pertinent to think of the NLRP3 inflammasome as a general sensor of cellular danger

TABLE 4.1 Selected Activators of the Inflammasome

NLRP1	NAIP/NLRC4	AIM2
Anthrax lethal toxin	Flagellin Bacterial type 3 secretion system proteins	dsDNA
	NLRP3	
Increased extracellular ATP Potassium efflux Calcium imbalance Osmotic change and cell swelling Mitochondrial DNA Beta amyloid plaque UV radiation	Nigericin Pore-forming toxins, e.g., hemolysin, pneumolysin, cholera toxin B Reactive oxygen species Cardiolipin Fatty acids and oxLDL Microbial nucleic acid	Lysosomal leakage Cholesterol crystals Alum Silica Uric acid Thioredoxin-interacting protein Fungal beta glucans

and perturbed homeostasis, i.e., a broad wide-ranging immune sensor that plays a critical role in driving cellular inflammation.

The inflammasome is a proinflammatory complex and therefore requires tight regulation as inappropriate activation has the potential to lead to unnecessary and potentially harmful inflammation. The impact of this is clearly seen when considering the role of the inflammasome in autoinflammatory disorders (Section 6.4). Consequently, there are a wide range of mechanisms employed to regulate inflammasome activity and some of these are introduced in Section 4.2.3. However, of particular relevance to the activation of inflammasome signaling is the concept of receptor autoinhibition.

In the absence of ligand stimulation the NLR inflammasome sensor proteins are kept in an inactive conformation in which the protein binds to ADP and the C-terminal leucine-rich repeats (LRRs) fold over and interact with regions of the central NACHT domain. This stops the sensors from interacting with one another and therefore inhibits inflammasome assembly. The maintenance of the autoinhibited state may well be aided by the presence of chaperone proteins such as HSP70, HSP90, and SGT1. The replacement of ADP with ATP most likely loosens this conformation to allow the LRRs to recognize their ligand. This results in further conformational rearrangements in the sensor, which then allow protein:protein interactions to occur, position the CARD or Pyrin effector domains to enable interaction with the adaptor proteins, and initiate inflammasome complex formation. Mutations in the central region, often referred to as the NACHT domain, are able to disrupt formation of the autoinhibited complex, which can lead to chronic

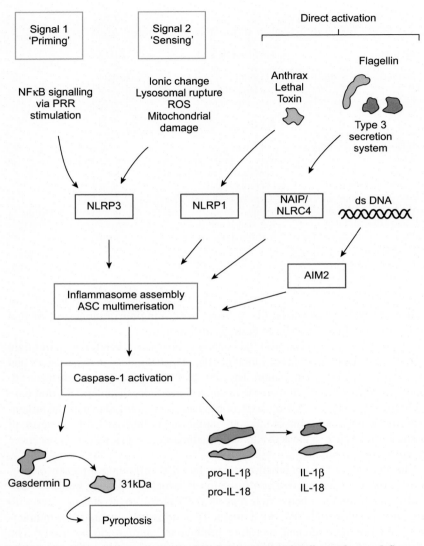

FIGURE 4.8 Schematic representation of the inflammasome signaling pathways. Inflamma-some sensors are activated by their ligands and initiate assembly of the inflammasome complex. NLRP3 requires both "priming," which follows from NFκB signaling, and a "sensing" step. NLRP1, NAIP/NLRC4, and AIM2 are directly activated by specific ligands. Activation of the sensor results in assembly of the inflammasome complex which includes multimerization of the adaptor ASC. This subsequently leads to caspase-1 activation, which then processes pro-IL-1β and pro-IL-18 to their active forms, and also cleaves Gasdermin D to create a 31 kDa fragment that drives cell death via pyroptosis. *ROS*, reactive oxygen species.

activation of the inflammasome and disease (Section 6.4). AIM2 also adopts an autoinhibited conformation in which its Pyrin domain is sequestered and unavailable to interact with the Pyrin domain of ASC. Binding of the AIM2 HIN200 domain to its dsDNA ligand releases the Pyrin domain and creates an active conformation.

4.2.1.1 The NLRP1 Inflammasome

Most of our understanding of the activation of the NLRP1 inflammasome comes from studies on murine NLRP1b, which detects the anthrax Lethal Toxin (LeTx). How relevant these are to human NLRP1 is questionable as while both the human and murine proteins contain a C-terminal CARD, human NLRP1 also contains a Pyrin domain in its N-terminal region, which is missing in the murine protein. The functional impact of this difference is unclear but may influence how the proteins interact with ASC.

The actual activation of the NLRP1b inflammasome is unusual in that the sensor protein, NLRP1b, has to be cleaved prior to activation. Cleavage occurs in two distinct places. One site is within the FIIND domain toward the C-terminus of the protein, and this happens in an autocatalytic manner. The second site occurs in the unstructured N-terminus and is actually brought about by the action of the anthrax LeTx. This raises the possibility that NLRP1b may not recognize LeTx directly via binding to the NLRP1b LRRs, but that it may in fact be a substrate for the toxin, which processes NLRP1b to drive activation, inflammasome assembly, and inflammatory signaling. If this is the case it raises the obvious possibility that other proteases, of host or pathogen origin, could also cleave and therefore activate NLRP1b. The human protein has not yet been shown to be a target for cleavage. Instead it is postulated to recognize the bacterial peptidoglycan fragment muramyl dipeptide (MDP), though this may occur in a manner dependent on the bona fide MDP sensor NOD2.

4.2.1.2 The NAIP/NLRC4 Inflammasome

The NAIP/NLRC4 inflammasome recognizes and interacts directly with bacterial flagellin and components of the bacterial type III secretion system apparatus. Members of the NAIP family function as the sensor, which then activates NLRC4 to enable inflammasome activation. The NAIP/NLRC4 and the NLRP1 inflammasomes have both been shown by electron microscopy to form wheel-like structures in the early stages of formation of the inflammasome complex. This process is described in more detail in Section 4.3.6.

4.2.1.3 The AIM2 Inflammasome

Formation of the AIM2 inflammasome is stimulated by the presence of dsDNA fragments at least 80 nucleotides long in the cellular cytoplasm. There is no sequence specificity to the recognition of dsDNA by AIM2; it is instead driven entirely by electrostatic charged–based interactions. In particular, positively charged amino acids located in the nucleic acid binding OB-folds of the AIM2 HIN200 domain interact with the negatively charged phosphate groups of the DNA (Fig. 4.9). This process releases AIM2 from its autoinhibited state by freeing the Pyrin domain. AIM2 forms oligomers along the DNA sequence and this may function as a switch for activation. On DNA sequences shorter than 80 nucleotides, insufficient AIM2 is recruited to overcome the activation threshold required to allow its Pyrin domain to act as a nucleation point for the recruitment, polymerization, and subsequent filament formation of ASC. Consistent

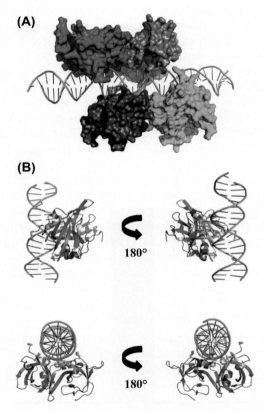

FIGURE 4.9 AIM2 binds dsDNA using its HIN200 domain. The HIN200 domain of AIM2 forms contacts with both the major and minor grooves of its dsDNA target. Binding between the HIN200 domain and the dsDNA leads to the formation of aggregates of AIM200 (A). In this panel the HIN200 domains are shown in surface representation and colored differently to show that they are derived from separate AIM2 proteins. (B) The interaction between AIM2 and dsDNA involves mainly basic residues on the AIM2 surface (K160, K162, K163, K198, K204, R244, K251, L267, N287, K309, R311, K335, I337, and K340). These are shown in *stick* representation, colored green, and presented from side-on (top panel) and end-on perspectives. The figures were generated from the PDB 3RN5.

with its different domain structure–Pyrin:HIN200—in comparison with the NLRs—Pyrin/CARD:NACHT:LRRs—there is no evidence that AIM200 forms wheel-like structures similar to those observed for NLRP1 and NAIP/NLRC4. Consequently, although the general biological function of the AIM2 inflammasome is the same as an NLR-driven inflammasome (caspase-1 activation, IL-1β and IL-18 production), the initial molecular interactions driving inflammasome formation are somewhat different between the two sensor systems.

4.2.1.4 The NLRP3 Inflammasome

The activation of the aforementioned inflammasomes is essentially a one-step process driven by the recognition of ligand, which facilitates the conformational rearrangements necessary to allow inflammasome assembly, caspase-1 activation, and the processing of pro-IL-1β and pro-IL-18. In contrast, straight exposure of cells to an NLRP3 inflammasome activator tends not to lead to the release of significant levels of IL-1β. This is because NLRP3 activation is a two-stage process. These stages are commonly referred to as "signal 1" and "signal 2," or "priming" and "sensing" (Fig. 4.8).

Signal 1, or priming, occurs upon the exposure of cells to PAMPs, DAMPs, or other stimuli that initiate NFκB-driven signaling pathways. Activation of PRR signaling pathways, particularly the TLR pathways, is therefore a major route of NLRP3 inflammasome priming. In experimental systems, priming usually occurs through the administration of extracellular LPS and the subsequent activation of TLR4 signaling. The key transcriptional changes that occur during priming are increases in the expression of the *NLRP3*, *IL1B*, and *IL18* genes. This is followed by increased rates of translation of the NLRP3 and pro-IL-1β proteins. Consequently, the levels of these proteins are increased in the cell and then permit the subsequent formation and function of the NLRP3 inflammasome. As stated earlier, this priming step is not necessary for the other types of inflammasome, the activation thresholds of which are presumably not limited by the levels of sensor proteins constitutively present in the cell. However, in the presence of high concentrations of suitable "priming" stimuli, each of these inflammasomes does appear to function more efficiently. This effect might well be due to simple reaction kinetics as a result of the increased levels of substrate available for processing.

Signal 2, or sensing, is the process by which the NLRP3 inflammasome is actually switched on and moves from a state of readiness to a state of activation and leads to assembly of the macromolecular inflammasome complex. It happens as a result of the presence of a suitable activatory ligand, such as one among those listed in Table 4.1. Given that these ligands are unlikely, or in some cases unable, to interact directly with NLRP3, it is most likely that NLRP3 "senses" some form of cellular perturbation or homeostatic change. A number of potential trigger processes have been described, which include osmotic imbalance, lysosomal leakage and disruption, reactive oxygen species

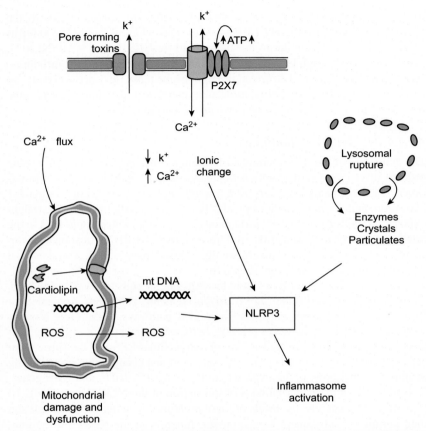

FIGURE 4.10   Schematic overview of the different ways that the NLRP3 "senses" danger during signal 2. Multiple indicators of cellular stress, damage, and homeostatic disruption are "sensed" by the NLRP3 inflammasome. These include changes in ion concentration, particularly in K$^+$ and Ca^{2+}; rupture and release of the contents of lysosomes; and damage to mitochondria that can increase reactive oxygen species (ROS) production, release mitochondrial DNA into the cytoplasm, and lead to a relocation of cardiolipin to the outer mitochondrial membrane.

(ROS) production, mitochondrial damage, and ionic efflux (Fig. 4.10). These processes are not necessarily mutually exclusive, may all have a role to play, and may ultimately turn out to precipitate a common cellular change that serves as the definitive trigger for NLRP3 inflammasome activation.

Significant cellular damage, particularly if it disrupts calcium signaling, often results in damage to the mitochondria. The precise role of the mitochondria in NLRP3 activation remains an uncertain, and to an extent a controversial, area of inflammasome biology. There has always been an interest in the connection between mitochondria and the NLRP3 inflammasome, both as a source of NLRP3 activators and also as a site for assembly of the actual inflammasome complex. Mitochondrial DNA, the mitochondrial phospholipid cardiolipin, the redox regulator thioredoxin interacting protein, and ROS generated in the mitochondria, have all been suggested to function as direct ligands for NLRP3. However, given their molecular differences, this is unlikely. It is clear that at least in some form or other, damaged mitochondria lead to NLRP3 activation. Precisely what the actual connection between mitochondria and the NLRP3 inflammasome is remains to be clarified.

Another cellular organelle proposed to activate the NLRP3 inflamma-some is the lysosome. It is clear that both particulate and crystalline materials (Table 4.1) can stimulate NLRP3 activation following their uptake by macro-phages. The phagocytosis of particulate and crystalline material can be prob-lematic for the macrophage, both in terms of the size of the molecule and in its relatively stable and inert composition. These attributes make crystalline mate-rial exceptionally difficult to break down and degrade. Consequently a common side effect of the phagocytosis of these materials is the rupture of the lysosomes in which they are contained. The lysosome is home to a harsh physiochemical environment, as well as a range of degrading enzymes such as members of the Cathepsin proteases. Therefore the release of the lysosomal contents into the cytoplasm has the potential to cause significant damage. However, many of the ligands that activate NLRP3, including ATP and various pore-forming bacterial toxins, do not get phagocytosed, do not come into contact with lysosomes, and do not lead to the release of lysosomal contents into the cytoplasm. Therefore, while lysosomal leakage may well trigger the activation of the NLRP3 inflam-masome, it is most certainly not the only trigger. In vaccine formulations in which alum is the adjuvant, and diseases involving crystalline or particulate components such as gout and atherosclerosis, lysosomal rupture–mediated NLRP3 activation may well be a major pathological driving force (see Sections 5 and 6).

A common side effect of cellular damage and homeostatic disruption is alteration of the ionic balance. This is often caused by changes in calcium and potassium signaling and may result from changes in ion storage, or in the activity of ion transporters leading to the efflux, or influx, of ions into the cytoplasm. Increasing calcium concentration can activate NLRP3, though this of course may be the result of associated damage to mitochon-dria. In contrast, it is the efflux of potassium that is connected with the NLRP3 inflammasome. Some of the earliest studies suggested that potas-sium efflux is the driving force behind inflammasome activation, and this theory has recently regained popularity as it is proposed to be a unifying cellular change that occurs in response to all NLRP3 stimuli, whether these result in (or from) mitochondrial damage, lysosomal rupture, or some other form of homeostatic imbalance. At the mechanistic level, potassium efflux can be brought about by the direct formation of pores in the plasma mem-brane as occurs with numerous bacterial pore-forming toxins; through the action of ionophores such as the widely used NLRP3 activator Nigericin;

and following activation of P_2X_7 purinergic receptors, which is brought about by high concentrations of ATP. It may well be that potassium efflux is a common theme in NLRP3 inflammasome activation, however, as yet how a reduction in potassium concentration would initiate the actual assembly of the inflammasome complex has not been investigated. The most likely scenario is that the change in ionic concentration causes a conformational rearrangement in NLRP3 that stops autoinhibition and permits protein:protein interactions to drive complex formation.

4.2.2 Protein Interactions Drive Assembly of the Inflammasome

The NLR proteins that act as sensors of the inflammasome are very similar in their domain organization to Apaf-1, which recognizes cytochrome c released from damaged mitochondria and interacts with pro-caspase-9 to initiate apoptosis. In the process of doing this, Apaf-1 forms a wheel-like structure, known as the apoptosome, containing seven Apaf-1 proteins. The view has long been held therefore that the inflammasome sensors will form similar wheel-like structures, and this does at least appear to be the case for NLRP1 and NAIP/NLRC4, albeit with a different stoichiometry to that seen for the apoptosome. In addition to ligand recognition, ATP binding appears to be a crucial step in allowing complex formation. Within these complexes, each individual protein interacts with its binding partners via interactions between the central NACHT domains, leaving the effector CARD or Pyrin domains available to interact with one another and with adaptor proteins to drive the overall formation of the resultant inflammasome.

The CARD and the Pyrin are both members of the Death Domain protein superfamily. Just as with formation of the Myddosome, the macromolecular complex essential for signaling downstream of TLRs (Section 2.2.4), death domains are the key protein fold in inflammasome assembly. The solved structures of Pyrin and CARD domains relevant to the assembly of the inflammasome complex are shown in Fig. 4.11. These domains interact with themselves and with one another in a homotypic manner (i.e., Pyrin with Pyrin, CARD with CARD) to facilitate the formation of the final inflammasome structure. For example, the Pyrin domain of NLRP3 binds the Pyrin domain of ASC, which then uses further Pyrin:Pyrin interactions to recruit more ASC and form a filamentous structure. These filaments act as a site for the recruitment of pro-caspase-1 via interactions between the CARD of ASC and the CARD of pro-caspase-1 (Fig. 4.12). Studies using cryoelectron microscopy have dramatically advanced our understanding of these interactions and indicate that they involve the classical Type I, II, and III death domain interaction surfaces (Section 2.2.4). These interactions are often dominated by surface charge, but also involve hydrophobic contacts. The formation of the Pyrin and CARD filaments generally requires a nucleating surface and, for example, both the NLRP3 and the ASC Pyrin can act as the nucleation point for ASC filament formation (Fig. 4.12).

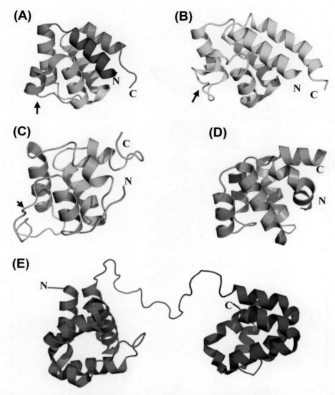

FIGURE 4.11 Pyrin domain and caspase recruitment domain (CARD) structures involved in inflammasome formation. Consistent with their classification as members of the Death Domain superfamily, the Pyrin domain and CARDs adopt a six-helix bundle structure. Pyrin domains are shown for (A) Human NLRP3 (PDB 3QF2), (B) Murine AIM2 (PDB 2N00), and (C) Human NLRP1 (PDB 1PN5). The N and C termini of the domain are labeled and in the case of the human NLRP3 in panel A the structure is colored from blue at the N-terminus to red at the C-terminus. The human NLRP1 Pyrin domain (C) lacks the third helix (position marked by an arrowhead), which is also heavily truncated in the AIM2 Pyrin domain (B). This probably influences functional interactions of the proteins. (D) The CARD of human NLRP1 (PDB 3KAT) and (E) full-length ASC showing both the Pyrin domain (red) and the CARD (blue) connected by a flexible linker (gray) that permits free movement of the domains and allows them to function independently of one another. The orientations of the proteins in panels A–D are identical.

4.2.3 Regulation of the Inflammasome Is Important

The importance of inflammasome regulation, the concurrent control of its pro-inflammatory signaling, and the presence of autoinhibited conformations for the sensor proteins has already been alluded to. There are many diverse ways in which the functionality of the inflammasome can be controlled to ensure that it is only activated under the most appropriate circumstances. Of courses these processes, while in some instances sharing an element of redundancy, are not foolproof and do sometimes fail, particularly in the face of genetic mutation.

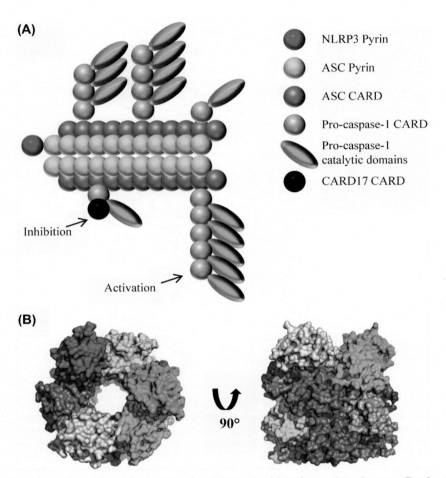

FIGURE 4.12 **Inflammasome assembly involves multiple interactions between Death Domain family members.** (A) Schematic representation of the interactions between the Pyrin domains and caspase recruitment domains (CARDs) in the assembly of the inflammasome. The NLRP3 Pyrin domain (*red sphere*) interacts with the ASC Pyrin domain (*gold sphere*) and acts as a nucleation point for ASC filament formation, which is driven by homotypic interactions between ASC Pyrin domains. The ASC CARD (*blue sphere*) points out of the filament and recruits the CARD of pro-caspase-1 (*lilac sphere*). This brings the pro-caspase-1 catalytic domains (*green ovals*) into close proximity with one another, allowing them to autocatalytically activate and release the catalytic domains to target substrates such as pro-IL-1β and pro-IL-18. Recruitment of CARD17 (*black sphere*) to the pro-caspase-1 filament inhibits caspase activation. (B) Cryoelectron microscopy studies highlight the multiinterface nature of the ASC filament. Each different color represents a different ASC Pyrin domain. Images generated from PDB 3J63.

Posttranslational modifications, particularly in the form of phosphorylation and ubiquitination, play an important role in the regulation of inflammasome activation. Phosphorylation can be used to both permit and inhibit inflammasome-related signaling events. This is best demonstrated through the phosphorylation of ASC, which most likely comes about through kinase pathways dependent on either Syk or Jnk. In murine ASC, phosphorylation of Ser144 positively regulates signaling. This modification is necessary for assembly of the full inflammasome complex and also regulates additional phosphorylation events on ASC. In contrast, addition of a phosphate to Ser293 in ASC by IKKα stops inflammasome signaling as a result of causing ASC to be retained in the nucleus. Consistent with its ability to signal independently of ASC, changes in ASC phosphorylation do not significantly influence NAIP/NLRC4 signaling. However, the activity of the NAIP/NLRC4 inflammasome is affected by phosphorylation of Ser533 in NLRC4 which, at least in some cell types, appears to be important for permitting downstream signaling events. Phosphorylation at Ser533 of NLRC4 is probably carried out by protein kinase C delta.

Ubiquitination involves the addition of small ubiquitin protein molecules either individually or in linear chains to the target protein. Depending on how the ubiquitin is linked, this can have a range of physiological functions and may act as a steric block of protein interactions, create an interface to permit recruitment of binding partners, or signal for protein degradation. Ubiquitination is important for the priming stage of NLRP3 inflammasome activation. The increased levels of NLRP3 protein produced as a result of priming only become competent for activation and assembly once they have been deubiquitinated. ASC is also regulated by ubiquitination, with the inflammasome failing to form if deubiquitination of ASC is inhibited. Meanwhile the AIM2 inflammasome can be marked for degradation via the addition of ubiquitin complexes.

The inflammasome can also be regulated by the action of specific regulatory proteins. These come in many shapes and sizes but include Pyrin-only and CARD-only proteins, which are known as POPs and COPs, respectively. These proteins consist of either just a Pyrin domain or a CARD and are capable of interacting with other Pyrin domains or CARDs involved in inflammasome assembly. In some instances, they are the result of duplications of portions of genes such as those encoding the ASC or AIM2 Pyrin domain or caspase-1 CARD. POP2, which is highly similar to the Pyrin domains of NLRP2 and NLRP7, interacts with the ASC Pyrin domain and interferes with inflammasome formation and function. POP3, on the other hand, is most similar to the AIM2 Pyrin domain and has been shown to interfere with the function of the AIM2, but not the NLR-initiated, inflammasome. In a similar vein the COPs CARD16, CARD17, and CARD18 are all able to interfere with caspase-1 processing, but only CARD17 appears to do this in the context of inflammasome signaling. In this instance CARD17 substitutes into growing filaments of caspase-1 and causes the termination of filament extension and subsequently stops caspase-1 from being activated (Fig. 4.12).

The NLRP3 inflammasome has also been shown to be inhibited by the naturally occurring ketone metabolite β-hydroxybutyrate at physiologically relevant concentrations in the range of 5–10 mM. Whether a much broader repertoire of endogenous metabolites exist, which have the capability of regulating NLRP3, or indeed other, inflammasomes remains to be seen.

4.3 THE INNATE RESPONSE TO BACTERIAL INFECTION WITH *SALMONELLA*

Pathogens represent a major threat to the host, and a large proportion of our immune repertoire has evolved to counter this threat. Exposure to pathogens such as the bacterium *Salmonella* requires a coordinated immune response and, in light of the wide range of immunostimulatory ligands it possesses, involves a variety of immune pathways working together and in parallel to fight infection.

4.3.1 Salmonellosis

Intestinal pathogens present a major global health burden and encompass a wide range of viral, bacterial, and parasitic infections. *Salmonella* is a clinically and economically important Gram-negative rod-shaped bacterium that survives well in a range of environments—from a few weeks in arid conditions to a few months in water. *Salmonella* possess flagella and are therefore motile. Infection with *Salmonella* has the capability of inducing acute and systemic diseases, the nature and severity of which differs with the type of animal host. There are only two species of *Salmonella*—*Salmonella enterica* and *Salmonella bongori*—and almost all cases of disease result from infection with *S. enterica*, of which there are over 2500 different serovars. These serovars can be broadly split into three categories based around the host range and the nature of infection. These include (1) rare with a highly restricted host range and pattern of infection such as human typhoid fever caused by *S. enterica enterica* serovar Typhi; (2) host-restricted potentially systemic infections, e.g., serovar Dublin in cattle, and serovar Choleraesuis in pigs; (3) serovars with broad host specificity that usually cause acute, localized gastroenteritis. In humans *S. enterica* enteritidis and *S. enterica* Typhimurium are the two most important serovars. In an immunocompromised host, these mild localized infections retain the potential to become systemic.

Gastroenteritis that can be attributed to *Salmonella* is referred to as Salmonellosis and is one of the most common global foodborne diseases. It is estimated that tens of millions of cases occur worldwide on an annual basis; however, this is likely to be an underestimate as many cases will not lead to contact with healthcare professionals and hence will not be recorded. The onset of salmonellosis is generally between 12 and 36 h from bacterial ingestion. Symptoms usually consist of a fever, abdominal pains and diarrhea, nausea, and occasionally, vomiting. Disease in otherwise healthy individuals is not normally particularly harsh and patients recover rapidly. However, salmonellosis can be much more severe in populations at greater risk of dehydration such as the young, the old, and the immunocompromised. Mortality associated with salmonellosis is a more significant problem in the developing world and leads to greater than 100,000 deaths per year. Antibiotic treatment can be employed for systemic infections, but antibiotic-resistant strains are becoming more common. The major source of infection is through the consumption of contaminated food products, particularly egg, milk, poultry, and meats. Consequently the most successful interventions are public health and food hygiene controls to limit the acquisition and subsequent spread of the bacteria.

4.3.2 *Salmonella* Is Recognized by a Range of Innate Immune Components

Unsurprisingly, infection with *Salmonella* spp., given its mechanism of transmission, occurs mainly in the intestines. The bacterium is one of a few examples of invasive bacterial pathogens that actively invade and survive in target cells. Other examples include, but are not limited to, *Listeria*, *Shigella*, and *Mycobacterium tuberculosis*. The chemical and physical defenses of the intestinal system—stomach acid, bile salts, mucin, antimicrobial peptides, secretory IgA—all provide some degree of protection against the establishment of infection. Within the intestinal lining itself, intestinal epithelial cells provide a physical barrier that helps to limit the spread of infection and also play an important role in the activation of the innate response via PRR-mediated recognition of the bacteria. Bacterial uptake by macrophages (and to a lesser extent dendritic cells) results in the stimulation of a wide range of PRRs, presents the main site of bacterial propagation, and can also serve as a route to systemic infection. The extent of the inflammatory response to *Salmonella* is a key contributor to the severity of infection, and this is driven predominantly through the interactions between *Salmonella* and a range of PRRs.

As an actively invasive bacterium, *Salmonella* stimulates its uptake into target cells by a mechanism widely referred to as the "trigger" method of entry, which has broad parallels with phagocytosis stimulated through engagement of antibody-specific Fc receptors. This process is extremely rapid, ending only a few minutes after first contact is made between the cell and the bacteria, and is stimulated by pathogen-specific effector proteins that are actively injected into the target cell cytosol via the *Salmonella* type III secretion systems and stimulate cytoskeletal rearrangements that drive internalization (Fig. 4.13). These effector proteins are found mainly on a specific pathogenicity island known as SPI-1 and include members of the Sip and Sop families. Once the bacteria are inside the cell, they stay in the endocytic vesicle and use this as a site of replication. To optimize the environment, *Salmonella* secrete a range of proteins, this time found on a second pathogenicity island, SPI-2, to alter the environment of the endosome. This ultimately creates a niche for bacterial replication that is protected from host defenses. This vacuole is known as the *Salmonella*-containing vacuole, or SCV (Fig. 4.13).

Recognition of *Salmonella* by the innate immune response is principally driven through the action of multiple PRRs. These include TLR1, 2, 4, 5, and 9; AIM2; NLRC4/NAIP; NLRP3; NOD1; and NOD2. The major

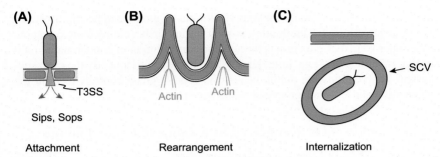

FIGURE 4.13 *Salmonella* **enters target host cells using the "trigger" method.** (A) *Salmonella* contact the surface of the target cell and inject effector proteins, such as Sops and Sips, which are encoded on the SPI-1 pathogenicity island, into the cytoplasm via a type 3 secretion system (T3SS, red). (B) The effector proteins stimulate rearrangement of the cytoskeleton, especially the actin component, to stimulate uptake of the bacteria. (C) The *Salmonella* bacterium is internalized into a vacuole. The subsequent expression of proteins from the SPI-2 pathogenicity island allows the bacteria to form a *Salmonella*-containing vacuole (SCV), in which it can survive and replicate.

Salmonella PAMPs that activate these PRRs are surface lipoproteins (TLR1, TLR2), LPS (TLR4), bacterial DNA (TLR9, AIM2), peptidoglycan (NOD1, NOD2), flagellin (TLR5, NLRC4/NAIP), and type III secretion system proteins (NLRC4/NAIP). A precise bacterial PAMP may activate the NLRP3 inflammasome, but it is more likely that this responds to the homeostatic disruption that results from infection with *Salmonella*. In addition, proteins such as caspase-4 (caspase-11 in rodents, caspase-13 in cows) also recognize *Salmonella*-derived LPS within the cytoplasm. Of these pathways the most crucial are those initiated via activation of TLR2, TLR4, TLR5, and NLRC4/NAIP.

We have already seen in Section 4.1 how TLR4 and inflammatory caspases recognize and respond to extracellular and intracellular LPS, respectively. Meanwhile Section 4.2 addresses the mechanisms by which the NLRP3 inflammasome can be activated to produce IL-1β. I will therefore focus the rest of this section on the innate response to *Salmonella* infection as mediated by activation of TLR2, TLR5, and the NLRC4/NAIP inflammasome.

4.3.3 *Salmonella*-Derived Lipoproteins Stimulate TLR2-Driven Inflammatory Signaling

TLR2 is a plasma membrane–bound PRR that recognizes acylated bacterial lipoproteins and signals as a heterodimer with either TLR1 or TLR6 (Fig. 4.14). The TLR2:TLR6 heterodimer is specific for diacylated lipoproteins, including lipoteichoic acid, which are found on Gram-positive bacteria. In contrast, the TLR2:TLR1 heterodimer is activated by triacylated lipoproteins derived from Gram-negative bacteria and is therefore the relevant system for the detection of *Salmonella*. These receptors can also be activated by the synthetic lipopeptides

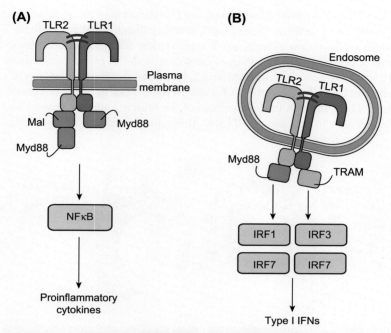

FIGURE 4.14   Schematic representation of the TLR2 signaling pathway. (A) The classical TLR2 signaling pathway involves activation at the plasma membrane and formation of a heterodimer with either TLR1 (shown) or TLR6. This permits recruitment of the adaptor proteins Mal and Myd88, formation of the Myddosome, and the production of proinflammatory cytokines in an NFκB-dependent manner. (B) More recently, it has been suggested that following activation the TLR2 heterodimer can be internalized to an endosome and signaling could be initiated from there. This leads type I interferon production via either IRF1 and IRF7 or IRF3 and IRF7 activation. The precise pathway depends on whether Myd88 or TRAM are recruited to the signaling complex.

Pam_3CSK_4 (triacylated—activates TLR1:TLR2) and Pam_2CSK_4 (diacylated—activates TLR2:TLR6).

At present the structure of TLR2:TLR1 in complex with a natural bacterial lipoprotein has not been solved. However, there is a good understanding of the molecular basis of ligand recognition because of the presence of structures for TLR2:TLR1 in complex with the triacylated synthetic ligand Pam_3CSK_4 and of TLR2:TLR6 in complex with Pam_2CSK_4, a diacylated ligand (Fig. 4.15). As with TLR4 the binding of ligand induces formation of an M-shaped complex involving two TLR molecules. However, unlike TLR4 the complexes of TLR2:TLR1 and TLR2:TLR6 only interact with a single ligand molecule, which serves to stabilize the formation of the M-shaped dimer (Fig. 4.15). In the case of the *Salmonella*-relevant TLR2:TLR1 heterodimer, this stabilization results from the binding of one amide-bound acyl chain into a hydrophobic pocket on TLR1 and two ester-bound acyl chains inserting into a hydrophobic pocket on TLR2 (Fig. 4.15).

As with TLR4-mediated signaling, the conformation of the receptors on the cell surface will facilitate the appropriate arrangement of the intracellular TIR domains to drive downstream signal transduction and proinflammatory cytokine production. TLR2 signaling is consistent with the broad mechanisms of TLR signaling described in Section 2.2.4 and can occur either as a result of direct interaction between the TLR2 and MyD88 TIRs or at lower concentrations of TLR2 through the engagement of the bridging adaptor protein Mal in a manner akin to that used by TLR4. Although the classic role for TLR2-led

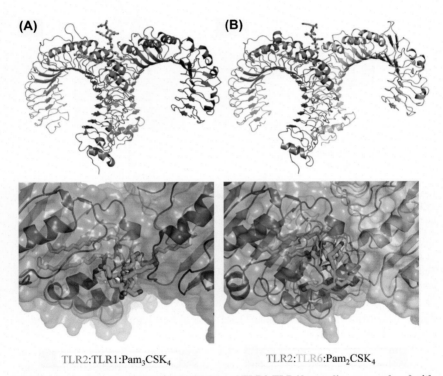

TLR2:TLR1:Pam$_3$CSK$_4$ TLR2:TLR6:Pam$_2$CSK$_4$

FIGURE 4.15 **Structures of the TLR2:TLR1 and TLR2:TLR6 heterodimers complexed with synthetic ligand.** The human TLR2:TLR1 (A) and murine TLR2:TLR6 (B) heterodimers both form classic M-shaped complexes with their triacylated (Pam$_3$CSK$_4$) and diacylated (Pam$_2$CSK$_4$) ligands, respectively. Only one ligand is found in each complex. Two acyl chains are inserted into a hydrophobic cavity in the TLR2 subunit. In addition the third acyl chain found in Pam$_3$CSK$_4$ inserts into a cavity in TLR1 and helps stabilize the complex. This cannot happen with the TLR2:TLR6 heterodimer because of the presence of two phenylalanine residues on TLR6 that block access to the pocket. Hence, TLR2:TLR6 binds diacylated ligands such as Pam$_2$CSK$_4$. TLR2 is colored slate blue, TLR1 raspberry red, and TLR6 orange. In the top panels, they are presented side-on in cartoon representation; the bottom panels are a top view to highlight the insertion of the acyl chains in the hydrophobic pockets. The ligand molecules are colored by atom type (green = carbon; blue = nitrogen; red = oxygen; yellow = sulfur). The images are generated from the PDB coordinate files 2Z7X (TLR2:TLR1) and 3A79 (TLR2:TLR6).

signaling is the formation of Myddosome complexes at the plasma membrane and the induction of NFκB signaling pathways, it is becoming apparent that, just like TLR4, TLR2-containing complexes can be endocytosed and then signal from the resulting endosome (Fig. 4.14). This process results in the production of IFN-β following recruitment of MyD88 and activation of IRF1 and IRF7. Endocytosed TLR2 complexes can also interact with the adaptor TRAM and initiate signaling pathway involving IRF3 and IRF7. It is not yet clear whether TLR2 signaling from the endosome is of relevance to the innate immune response to *Salmonella* infection.

4.3.4 Flagellin Is a Major Immune Stimulus

Salmonella are motile bacteria. This motility is provided by the presence of flagella. These drive both random tumbling and the directional movement toward food sources and chemoattractants and away from toxins and threats. *Salmonella* that have been genetically modified to either lack flagella or express nonfunctional variants are heavily impaired in their ability to establish infection. This is a result of a lack of contact between the bacteria and the cell as forced contact, for example, as a result of centrifugation, helps restore the ability of the bacteria to enter the target cells.

Bacterial flagella are filamentous proteins that extend around 20 nm from the surface of the bacterial cell. While relatively common on rod-shaped bacteria such as *Salmonella*, *E. coli*, and *Legionella pneumophila*, they are rarely found on cocci-shaped bacteria. The production of flagella is a complex process and involves approximately 50 separate genes to produce and assemble all the necessary components. The base of the flagella is anchored to the bacterial membrane through a structure known as the basal body formed from four distinct protein rings. In Gram-negative bacteria, two of these rings, S and M, are embedded in the inner plasma membrane, P is positioned in the periplasmic space, and L is found in the outer membrane. It is the innermost S and M rings that provide the rotational force for flagella movement. This rotation is powered chemiosmotically by the use of proton motive force. The basal body is attached to a hook structure, which in turn is attached to the filament that protrudes from the bacterium and provides motility upon rotation. The filament is formed by the polymerization of protein subunits. In the case of *Salmonella*, these subunits are known as flagellin and are encoded by the *FliC* gene. The outermost tip of the flagella is covered by a protein cap formed from FliD. It is the flagellin, i.e., the major constituent of the flagella filament, which is the major immunogenic component (Fig. 4.16).

4.3.5 Extracellular Flagellin Is Detected by TLR5

TLR5 is located in the plasma membrane of immune and nonimmune cells. It is particularly important in the maintenance of intestinal homeostasis. As such,

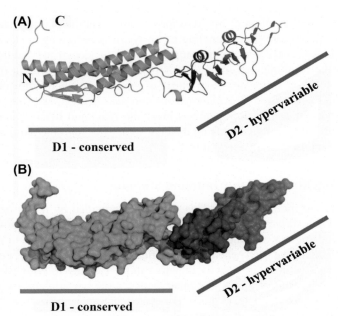

FIGURE 4.16 Structure of the FliC flagellin protein from *Salmonella*. (A) Cartoon and (B) surface representation of FliC, the major structural subunit of the *Salmonella* flagella. FliC is one of the primary immunostimulatory components of flagellated bacteria such as *Salmonella*. The D1 region of FliC (green) contains a stretch of highly conserved amino acids that are important for bacterial motility and the formation of the flagella filament. These residues are recognized by TLR5. The blue region, D2, is hypervariable and displays much sequence variation. Figure generated from PDB coordinate file 3V47. The N and C termini of the molecule are labeled in panel (A) and the orientation of both panels is the same.

higher levels of TLR5 are seen on the surface of mucosal macrophages and dendritic cells than on those found in other locations such as the spleen. TLR5 is also expressed in intestinal epithelial cells. To reduce the likelihood of inopportune or inappropriate activation, it is, however, localized to the basolateral (bottom), and not the apical (top), surface of these cells. This ensures that it only responds to the presence of flagellated bacteria that have breached the epithelial barrier. The absence of TLR5 in mice leads to alterations in the composition of the intestinal microbiota and leads to the development of physiological changes associated with metabolic syndrome and increased risk of conditions such as cardiovascular disease and type 2 diabetes.

Flagellin is detected directly by the LRRs of TLR5 (Fig. 4.17). Amino acids in the D1 region of flagellin (Fig. 4.16) form an extensive series of interactions with the first 10 LRRs of TLR5 (Fig. 4.17). Some bacteria such as *H. pylori* and *Campylobacter jejuni* possess flagella that are not recognized by TLR5, whereas flagellin from *Salmonella* is highly immunogenic. Comparing the flagellin sequences of these bacteria shows that nonimmunogenic flagellin has

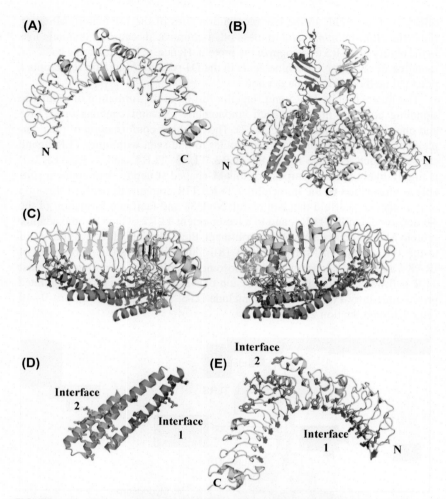

FIGURE 4.17 The structural basis of TLR5-mediated recognition of flagellin. (A) Cartoon representation of the ectodomain of zebrafish TLR5, which is composed of leucine-rich repeats (LRRs) and adopts a curved solenoid conformation. The C-terminal end is proximal to the surface of the host cell plasma membrane. (B) Signaling competent complex of two TLR5:FliC monomers coming together to form an M-shaped heterodimer. The left hand FliC molecule is colored green (D1) and blue (D2) as in panel (A). (C) Complex of FliC and TLR5 highlighting the two major interfaces between the D1 region of FliC and the TLR5 ectodomain. The major interface interactions involve residues from the first six TLR5 LRRs, whereas the second interface uses residues on LRR7-10. Both interfaces are mainly hydrophilic in nature. Interacting residues are represented as *sticks*. For clarity, only the three main helices of the FliC domain D1 are shown. Both panels are related by a 180 degrees rotation around the y axis. Interface 1 residues are colored blue (FliC) and brown (TLR5); interface 2 residues are cyan (FliC) and orange (TLR5). Interface residues for FliC (D) and TLR5 (E) are shown with the interfaces facing out of the page. Colors as in panel (C), figures generated from PDB coordinate file 3V47.

different amino acids in the key recognition sites of the D1 region. Mutating FliC (flagellin) in *Salmonella* to these other amino acids causes a dramatic loss in the ability of TLR5 to recognize the protein. Hence, at least for some bacteria, mutating or changing the amino acids in the D1 region of flagellin represents a practical method of immune evasion.

The interaction of TLR5 and flagellin results in the formation of a dimeric signaling complex in which each "monomeric" subunit contains one TLR5 and one flagellin molecule (Fig. 4.17). The resulting conformation of the complex has an M-shaped arrangement similar to that seen with other TLR-ligand structures such as those for TLR1:TLR2, TLR3, TLR4, and TLR6:TLR2. It is highly likely that the purpose of this M-shaped structure is to create a suitable conformation of the intracellular TLR5 TIR domains to permit formation of a molecular scaffold that can recruit MyD88 and facilitate formation of the Myddosome. Unlike TLR4, and to a lesser extent TLR2, which use the adaptor protein Mal to facilitate MyD88 recruitment, the TLR5 TIR directly binds itself to the TIR domain of MyD88 (Fig. 4 18). This then drives the recruitment of IRAK4 and IRAK1 to form the Myddosome complex and, common with most TLR pathways, results in the expression of NFκB and stress kinase regulated proinflammatory cytokines. These include IL-6, IL-12, TNFα, and pro-IL-1β (Fig. 4.18 and Section 2.2.4).

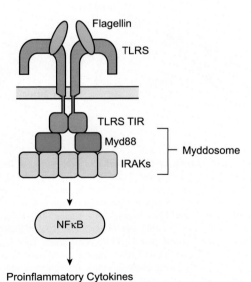

FIGURE 4.18 Schematic overview of the TLR5 signaling pathway. TLR5 signaling begins at the plasma membrane following the recognition of bacterial flagellin and the formation of a 2:2 complex of TLR5 and flagellin. The adaptor protein Myd88 is recruited directly to the TIR domains of TLR5, from which it drives the formation of a macromolecular Myddosome complex involving the IRAKs. This then activates NFκB-driven proinflammatory cytokine expression.

4.3.6 Intracellular Flagellin and Components of the Type III Secretion System Activate the NAIP/NLRC4 Inflammasome

Until recently the multiprotein complex activated by bacterial flagellin was referred to as the NLRC4 inflammasome as it had long been known that NLRC4 was essential for the intracellular detection of flagellin and the subsequent assembly of the caspase-1–activating inflammasome complex. This process was assumed to be driven by a direct interaction between NLRC4 and flagellin. Researchers were aware that the NAIPs were important for the activation of this inflammasome complex, but the molecular basis for this was unclear. Since 2011, it has become apparent that it is in fact the NAIP proteins that function as the sensors of bacterial flagellin—they also detect the needle and rod proteins of the bacterial type III secretion system. The NAIPs interact directly with the stimulatory ligand, before then binding NLRC4 to initiate inflammasome assembly (Fig. 4.19). Hence the complex is commonly now referred to as the NAIP/NLRC4 inflammasome. Within this complex the NAIPs act as the sensor protein and NLRC4 serves an adaptor protein function to recruit pro-caspase-1 and under some circumstances, ASC.

As with many of the studies performed to investigate the molecular basis of immune function, the majority of work investigating the NAIP/NLRC4 inflammasome has been performed using murine models and cells derived from mice. This is particularly important in this context as the genetics of the NAIP proteins are considerably different between mice and humans. Humans produce just a single full-length NAIP, whereas mice encode four functional NAIPs— NAIP1, NAIP2, NAIP5, and NAIP6. In mice each of these proteins appears, at least for now, to recognize a single type of ligand. NAIP1 is sensitive to the needle proteins in bacterial type III secretion systems; NAIP2 also responds to the type III secretion system, but in this case to the rod proteins (PrgJ in *Salmonella*); whereas both NAIP5 and NAIP6 seem to only be activated by the major component of bacterial flagella, i.e., FliC in *Salmonella*. Much of the early work seemed to ignore the question of whether human NAIP performed the role of all four of the murine NAIPs, or whether other alternative detection mechanisms might exist. However, it is now apparent that, at least in the case of macrophages, both bacterial flagella and proteins from the type III secretion system are able to activate human NAIP. This in itself raises intriguing questions about the selection pressures that have led to this alternative approach to the primary detection event.

The interaction between the NAIPs and their ligands appears to require helical regions with the central NACHT domain. It is not known yet whether this is a direct physical interaction, but at the mechanistic level, it seems to contrast with many other LRR-containing proteins, including the TLRs, in which it is the LRRs that interact directly with the activating ligand. Following ligand detection the NAIPs act as a nucleation point for oligomerization of NLRC4 and inflammasome formation. The early stages of this process have been visualized

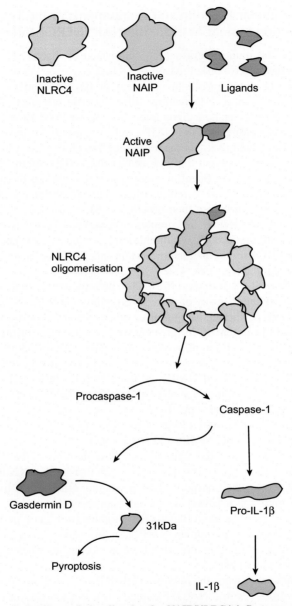

FIGURE 4.19 **Activation and signaling by the NAIP/NLRC4 inflammasome.** NAIP and NLRC4 are believed to exist in the cytoplasm in an inactive conformation. NAIP acts as the sensor molecule and responds to the presence of cytoplasmic flagellin and type 3 secretion system proteins. Ligand-bound NAIP then acts as a nucleating point for the activation and oligomerization of NLRC4 into wheel-like structures. NLRC4 can directly recruit pro-caspase-1 via CARD–CARD interactions, which is then activated and can process Gasdermin D to initiate pyroptosis and leads to IL-1β production. ASC can also be recruited to NLRC4 and appears to improve the efficiency of signaling.

in vitro using both negative-stained and cryoelectron microscopy and reveal the presence of wheel-like structures. These complexes are analogous to those formed in vitro by NLRP1 and also the Apaf-I:pro-caspase-9 apoptosome structure that drives the apoptotic signaling path activated by the release of cytochrome c from mitochondria.

The NAIP/NLRC4 complexes visualized by electron microscopy have a diameter approaching 60 nm and contain between 10 and 12 "spokes" to each wheel. The activated NAIP contributes only one of these "spokes" and suggests that the NAIP-ligand interaction functions as a molecular switch to drive conformational change in NLRC4, which then permits NACHT–NACHT interactions that drive NLRC4 oligomerization and the formation of the larger wheel-like structures. The details of how these NLRC4-rich wheel-like structures assemble into the final macromolecular inflammasome complex that can be visualized in the cytoplasm remain to be fully mapped out. However, in some of the cryoelectron microscopy studies, larger helical filaments that may provide insight into this process have been observed. It also appears that in some cell types phosphorylation of NLRC4 at Ser533 is necessary for permitting this assembly process to occur.

The NAIP/NLRC4 inflammasome complex forms within minutes of *Salmonella* infection occurring, highlighting the rapid nature of this protective response. The final complex contains, at the very least, a NAIP, NLRC4, and pro-caspase-1. However, in reality things are often much more complex than this. Superresolution microscopy has shown that both flagellin- and *Salmonella*-activated complexes can also contain NLRP3 in addition to NLRC4, as well as different effector caspases. Although NLRC4 can directly recruit pro-caspase-1 through CARD:CARD interactions, the main inflammasome adaptor ASC is also commonly incorporated into the NAIP/NLRC4 inflammasome structure. It appears that the presence of ASC serves to increase the efficiency of pro-caspase-1 recruitment and activation and hence enhances IL-1β production. This may also relate to the different effector functions of the NAIP/NLRC4 inflammasome. Without doubt the NAIP/NLRC4 inflammasome is extremely important for the induction of pyroptosis (Section 3.5.4), particularly during the early stages of infection. This process may be particularly relevant in limiting the establishment of any infection. In cells that do not undergo rapid pyroptosis, the production of IL-1β becomes more important as the cell continues to battle infection and call upon other defense mechanisms. The additional involvement of ASC may help drive the switch between these processes.

4.4 INNATE RECOGNITION AND THE RESPONSE TO THE *INFLUENZA* VIRUS

Influenza A virus (IAV) is the major cause of the respiratory infection influenza. It is a member of the *Influenzavirus* genus within the *Orthomyxoviridae* family. Along with Influenza B and C, it is one of the three serotypes in this genus. IAV is an enveloped virus with a genome composed of eight separate ssRNA segments contained within a ribonucleoprotein (RNP) core. In total, these segments code for 11 distinct genes. IAV is a major global pathogen and infects around 100 million people each year. It is responsible for annual epidemics worldwide of severe respiratory disease. These epidemics result in severe illness for up to five million people and can lead to death in around 10% of these cases. Mortality is often associated with the acquisition of secondary bacterial infections. Consequently, the actual cause of death is often bacterial pneumonia. The ability of IAV to dramatically shift its antigenic status and for avian, human, and porcine strains to undergo recombination gives IAV the potential to cause global pandemics with high mortality rates. For example the 1918 Influenza pandemic, "Spanish influenza," caused more deaths than World War I did in the preceding four years. Consequently, IAV represents a realistic biological threat at the global level.

4.4.1 The Influenza A Virus Replication Cycle

The replication cycle of IAV is summarized in Fig. 4.20. IAV is a respiratory pathogen and is principally transmitted via respiratory aerosol following expulsion from infected individuals when they cough or sneeze. However, IAV can also survive on inanimate surfaces and hence transmission can occur because of viral transfer from contaminated surfaces. The epithelial cells of the entire respiratory tract—nasal airways, trachea, small airways, and lungs—represent the major target cells for IAV infection. Entry of IAV is mediated by interaction of the globular domain of the viral hemagglutinin (HA) protein (Fig. 4.21), which is found on the virion surface, with the terminal sialic acid residue on glycosylated proteins on the surface of the target cell. Avian IAV preferentially binds to sialic acid with an α2-3 linkage, whereas human IAV strains interact more efficiently with sialic acid possessing an α2-6 linkage. Additional binding also occurs between sialic acid and another viral surface protein, neuraminidase (NA) (Fig. 4.20).

Binding mediates endocytosis of the viral particle. As the resulting endosome acidifies, this causes a dramatic conformational change in the HA molecule that drives fusion of the viral and endosomal membranes. HA exists as a trimer in which each contributing monomer is formed from two disulphide linked chains—HA1 and HA2. Before acidification the HA trimer adopts a broadly cylindrical conformation in which a stem region, containing HA1 and HA2 residues, positions the globular head (composed entirely of HA1) distal to the virion surface where it can bind to and interact with sialic acid (Fig. 4.21). In this conformation the fusion peptide, which is part of HA2, is found buried in the interior of the molecule. In the endosome the decrease in pH causes the HA2 region to rearrange, which includes a 180 degrees inversion of the C-terminal region (Fig. 4.21), and extend the fusion peptide into the endosomal membrane. This creates a hemifusion intermediate, which then proceeds into a full pore. Following acidification of the viral core, brought about by the role of the IAV proton channel–forming protein M2, the viral RNP is released into

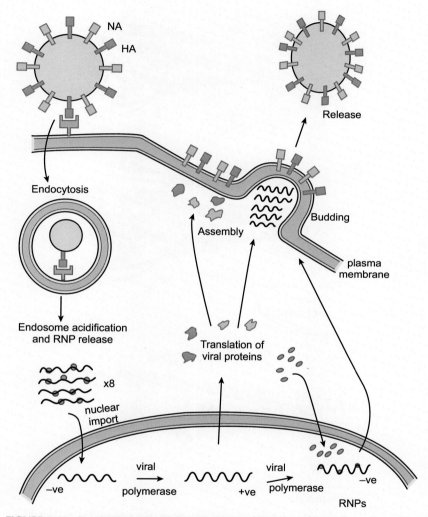

FIGURE 4.20 Replication cycle of the influenza A virus. Viral hemagglutinin (HA) on the surface of the virion particle interacts with sialic acid residues on host surface proteins triggering internalization. Acidification of the endosome causes HA-mediated membrane fusion and release of the viral ribonucleoproteins (RNPs) into the cytoplasm. These are imported into the nucleus and the viral RNA-dependent RNA polymerase makes new +ve and −ve sense RNA for use in translation and as new genomes. Virion assembly, budding, and release take place at the plasma membrane into which HA and neuraminidase (NA) have been inserted.

the cytoplasm (Fig. 4.20). Entry of the viral RNP into the nucleus is driven by nuclear localization signals present in the viral proteins NP, PA, PB1, and PB2 and happens in a Crm1-dependent manner. The negative sense ssRNA genome segments are then transcribed by the viral RNA-dependent RNA polymerase, which is formed from the viral proteins PA, PB1, and PB2. This requires the

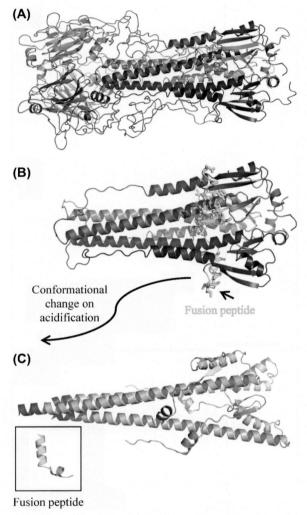

(A)

(B)

Conformational change on acidification

Fusion peptide

(C)

Fusion peptide

FIGURE 4.21 **Influenza A virus hemagglutinin is a critical viral protein.** (A) The global conformation of the influenza A virus hemagglutinin (HA) membrane protein. In this conformation the globular head (left) can interact with sialic acid residues on the surface of the target membrane and initiate viral entry. Each HA monomer is colored separately with the darker colors representing the HA2 chain and the lighter color the HA1 chain. The HA2 chain contains the fusion peptide. The virion membrane would be at the right of the image. (B and C) The HA2 domain alone of the HA protein in the preentry (B) and postendosome acidification (C) forms. Colors and orientation are the same as panel (A) but with the postendosome form (C) in a lighter shade. The extent of the conformational change in HA upon acidification is demonstrated by the reorganization of the HA2 fragment and movement of fusion peptide approximately 100 Å toward the host cell surface. The fusion peptide of each chain is displayed as *yellow sticks* in panel (B) and although not present in the structure of panel (C) is shown in its helical fusion form in the inset. The extent of the conformational change can be seen by comparing the position of the magenta sections in the pre- and postacidification forms, which represent the same amino acid sequence in HA2 in both panels. Figures were generated from PDB files 1HGE (Panels A and B), 1HTM (Panel C), and 1IBN (Panel C inset).

polymerase to "steal" 5′-cap structures from host RNAs. The resultant positive sense mRNA is then exported to the cytoplasm and used as a template for the translation of viral proteins (Fig. 4.20). The viral polymerase uses some of the positive ssRNA as a template for the production of more negative sense genomic RNA segments. These are bound by the viral NP protein, exported from the nucleus, and translocate to the cell membrane, where they associate with viral proteins and bud out of the infected cell. This new virion has HA and NA expressed on its surface as these proteins were inserted into the plasma membrane of the infected cell following their synthesis. The virion is now ready to locate and infect a new cell.

4.4.2 Antigenic Drift and Antigenic Shift in Influenza A Virus

There are 17 known subtypes of HA and 10 known subtypes of NA. These two proteins represent the major antigenic determinants of IAV and are the target of neutralizing antibodies produced from B cells, as part of the adaptive immune response. However, both HA and NA undergo antigenic changes to limit their immunogenicity and reduce, or neutralize, the effectiveness of the antibody-mediated host defenses. This occurs through two mechanisms, antigenic drift and antigenic shift, and are best understood in the context of HA.

Antigenic drift results from the incorporation of point mutations in the HA protein that alter the amino acid sequence and hence change the surface of the protein. These mutations occur because of the high rate of replication and the limited proof reading capacity of the viral RNA polymerase. They occur with the greatest frequency in the most antigenic regions of the protein (Fig. 4.21). The mutations serve to decrease the effectiveness of antibody recognition and binding and therefore decrease the usefulness of adaptive immune memory.

Antigenic shift results from genetic reassortment between two IAVs with different host specificity. In the context of human infection, it is most consequential when reassortment happens between either avian and human IAV, or porcine and human IAV. This process often occurs in a porcine host and requires coinfection of a single cell with the different viral strains. During packaging of the viral genome, different segment combinations are incorporated into the virion particles (Fig. 4.21). This can lead to the creation of viruses that are replication competent in human cells but possess avian or porcine HA or NA and hence are not recognized by the adaptive immune response. The host therefore acts as an immunologically naïve target resulting in rapid establishment of infection, high viral loads, and an excessive and potentially fatal inflammatory response.

4.4.3 Influenza A Virus and the Innate Immune Response

Infection of respiratory epithelial cells leads to the rapid induction of an innate immune response in the host. This results in the production of a variety of pro-inflammatory cytokines and chemokines including IL-6, IL-8, IL-1β, TNFα,

MCP1, CCL3, and CXCL10, as well as interferons and interferon-stimulated genes (ISGs). Both interferon production and ISG activation play an important role in the induction of an antiviral state in surrounding cells. MCP1 recruits monocytes and macrophages to the site of infection and activates them. Recognition of IAV is brought about by various PRRs, including members of the TLR, NLR, and RLR families.

IAV and TLRs: The recognition of IAV by members of the TLR family occurs within the endosome and is mainly driven by TLR7, which recognizes ssRNA. TLR3, which is activated by dsRNA, also responds to IAV infection, presumably as a result of detecting either replication intermediates or structured regions of the genome that lead to the formation of regions of dsRNA. The activation and signaling pathways of TLR3 have been described earlier in Section 2.2.4. TLR7, like TLR3, is an endosomally located PRR and also stimulates the production and secretion of antiviral type I interferons. However, the receptors rely mainly on the use of different transcription factors to achieve this—IRF3 in the case of TLR3 and IRF7 for TLR7. Detection of viral ssRNA activates TLR7 and facilitates recruitment of MyD88, formation of a Myddosome, and activation of IRF7 via a TRAF3 and IKKα-dependent pathway. TLR7 expression levels are highest in tissues and surfaces likely to come into contact with viral pathogens, consistent with their role in detecting viral infection. This includes the intestines and the lungs. TLR7 is also highly expressed in plasmacytoid dendritic cells, which are a major source of IFN production in the response to infection with IAV and other viruses.

IAV and RLRs: The RLR family member RIG-I is crucial to the specific innate response to IAV infection. MDA-5 in contrast, along with PKR, a dsRNA activated kinase, serves to enhance the generation of a more general antiviral state. RIG-I recognizes short 5′ tri- or diphosphorylated dsRNA sequences. Although the genome of IAV is single-stranded, it contains structured regions that lead to the formation of short stretches of dsRNA. In particular, partially complementary regions at the 5′ and 3′ ends of the viral genome segments form structures known as "panhandles," which contain stretches of dsRNA. These structures are known to be capable of activating RIG-I, as are double-stranded segments of defective interfering genome generated during replication by the viral polymerase switching between genome segments before transcription is complete. RIG-I also detects the viral RNP complexes released following fusion of the viral and endosomal membranes. None of these elements are present in the cytoplasm of uninfected cells, thereby ensuring that activation of RIG-I is virus specific and not the result of inappropriate detection of host RNA.

The molecular basis of RIG-I activation has been well documented and a series of structural studies have provided clear insight into how the RNA ligand is recognized, the conformational changes this induces in RIG-I, and how this facilitates downstream signal transduction to drive RIG-I–mediated immunity.

RIG-I is composed of two N-terminal CARDs, a DExD/H-helicase domain and a C-terminal domain (CTD). In the absence of suitable ligand, RIG-I adopts a closed conformation in which the CARDs are sequestered as a result of inter-action with the helicase domain and are unable to interact with downstream sig-naling partners (Fig. 4.22). RIG-I has a very low threshold of activation, and the presence of just 20 suitable dsRNA ligands is sufficient to stimulate RIG-I acti-vation and signaling. Binding initially occurs between the CTD of RIG-I and the RNA ligand (Fig. 4.22), which stimulates extensive conformational changes

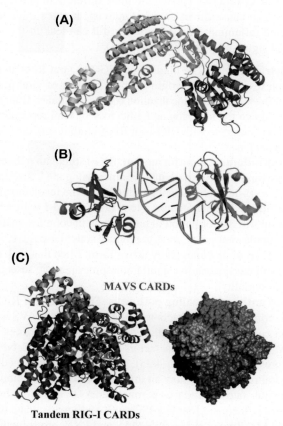

FIGURE 4.22 **The structural basis of RIG-I activation.** (A) Overall structure of RIG-I from the mallard duck (PDB 4A2W) showing the discrete domain organization in the inactive confor-mation. CARD 1 (light orange), CARD 2 (dark orange), helicase domain 1 (raspberry), helicase domain 2 (gold), helicase insertion domain (light blue), bridging domain (magenta). The C-terminal domain (CTD) was unstructured and not visible in this X-ray structure. (B) The CTD of RIG-I bound to a fragment of dsRNA (PDB 4A2X). The short dsRNA fragment is bound by two discrete CTDs, one colored red and one blue. (C) The complex formed between the caspase recruitment domains (CARDs) of RIG-I and MAVS to drive RIG-I mediated signaling (PDB 4P4H). The tan-dem RIG-I CARDs are colored in shades of blue, the MAVS CARD in shades of red. The side view is in cartoon representation, whereas the top view, a surface representation. Further recruitment of MAVS CARD leads to filament formation.

that result in further interactions occurring between the helicase domain and the RNA molecule. The helicase–RNA interactions are not sequence specific because they occur mainly with the sugar-phosphate backbone (Fig. 4.22). This process serves to release the CARD domains from their autoinhibited conformation and allows them to be targeted for K63-linked polyubiquitination by the E3 ligase TRIM25, which sets them up for interaction with other CARDs, such as those in MAVS, to initiate antiviral signaling and innate defenses.

Activation of RIG-I by IAV can lead to three different innate immune effector responses. It can cause direct antiviral activity; it can stimulate formation of a noncanonical inflammasome structure; and it can lead to the induction of specific antiviral signaling pathways (Fig. 4.23).

- **Direct antiviral activity**: The binding of RIG-I to viral RNA in the released vRNP complexes serves to interfere with the binding of viral proteins to the RNA and inhibits the nuclear localization of these particles. Both these effects serve to slow down the initiation and efficiency of viral replication. The IAV protein NS1 can compete with RIG-I for RNA binding and therefore limit the impact of this defense.

- **Noncanonical inflammasome formation**: RIG-I stimulation induces multiple signaling pathways. One of these involves increasing the transcription of pro-IL-1β in an NFκB-dependent manner but without the involvement of MAVS, CARD9, or Bcl10. The subsequent interaction of RIG-I with ASC and pro-caspase-1 results in the formation of a multiprotein complex analogous to the classical inflammasomes that serves to produce active caspase-1, which in turn cleaves pro-IL-1β to its biologically active form. Mice that lack components required to form this noncanonical inflammasome are more susceptible to IAV infection and mortality.

- **Activation of antiviral signaling pathways**: The CARDs of RIG-I can form a tetrameric complex that interacts with the CARDs of MAVS and serves as a nucleation center for the formation of filamentous structures. These lead to the activation of transcription factors such as IRF3 and NFκB and the ultimate expression of ISGs (Fig. 4.23). These ISGs are key mediators of the innate antiviral response and play an important role in the establishment of a cellular antiviral state that reduces permissiveness to infection. In the context of IAV infection, there are four key ISGs—2′-5′-oligoadenylate (OAS), PKR, IFITM3, and Mx. Two of these, 2′-5′-OAS and PKR, are sometimes thought of as intracellular PRRs. They both recognize dsRNA and in the case of 2′-5′-OAS stimulate synthesis of RNAse L, which degrades the viral genome, whereas PKR activates NFκB, recruits RLRs, and inhibits viral translation. IFITM3 and Mx interfere with IAV entry into the host cell and import of the vRNP into the nucleus respectively.

IAV and NLRs: The NLRs are not principally associated with the detection of viral infection. However, the disruption of cellular homeostasis that occurs upon IAV infection is sufficient to stimulate activation of the NLRP3 inflammasome and the production of IL-1β and IL-18. The mechanistic basis behind IAV-driven activation of NLRP3 has not been fully defined, but viral ssRNA, the M2 ion-channel forming protein, and lysosomal aggregation of the IAV protein PB1-F2 have all been put forward as NLRP3 activators. A comprehensive description of NLRP3 activation and signaling is provided in Section 4.2.

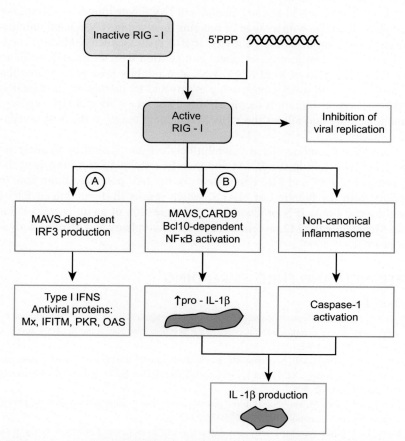

FIGURE 4.23 Downstream signaling pathways and effector functions induced by RIG-I activation. (A) RIG-I activation by dsRNA causes the production of type I interferons and the upregulation of antiviral molecules. Recognition of ligand releases RIG-I from its inactive state and permits interaction between the caspase recruitment domains (CARDs) of RIG-I and MAVS, which is attached to the mitochondrial membrane. This leads to the ultimate activation of IRF3 and the subsequent production of antiviral molecules and type I interferons. (B) RIG-I can upregulate NFκB pathways via MAVS, CARD9, and Bcl10 to increase levels of pro-IL-1β and also form a noncanonical inflammasome through association with ASC and pro-caspase-1. This leads to caspase-1 activation and increased IL-1β production. (C) RIG-I can also interfere with viral replication by binding to the viral RNA and encouraging disassembly of viral protein complexes.

4.4.4 Evasion of the Innate Immune Response by Influenza A Virus

The processes of antigenic drift and shift have been briefly described earlier. These two processes are critical immune evasion tools, but function against the adaptive and not the innate immune response. As with many viral infections, particularly the most successful ones, IAV has a wide repertoire of innate immune evasion strategies.

The viral protein NS1 is a key mediator of IAV innate immune evasion. For example, it interacts with a range of proteins involved in IFN-related immune defenses and neutralizes their activity. It also possesses RNA binding capabilities and can therefore act in direct competition with TLRs and RIG-I to inhibit the detection of viral RNA. NS1 also inhibits host gene expression by interfering with mRNA processing events and by disrupting the function of the translation initiation factor eIF4B. This serves to globally suppress immune activity and allows the virus to dominate usage of the host translational machinery.

The IAV polymerase can also inhibit host cell translation by stealing the cap complexes from host mRNAs and therefore stopping recruitment of the ribosome. The PB1 and PB2 components of the IAV polymerase are able to interfere with the function of MAVS, which results in disruption of RIG-I signaling and limits IFN production and the creation of an antiviral cellular state. Meanwhile the M2 protein disrupts host autophagy and disrupts activation of PKR.

REFERENCES AND FURTHER READING

Section 4.1

Aglietti RA, Estevez A, Gupta A, Ramirez MG, Liu PS, Kayagaki N, et al. GsdmD p30 elicited by caspase-11 during pyroptosis forms pores in membranes. Proc Natl Acad Sci USA June 23, 2016;113(28):7858–63.

Bryant CE, Orr S, Ferguson B, Symmons MF, Boyle JP, Monie TP. International union of basic and clinical pharmacology. XCVI. Pattern recognition receptors in health and disease. Pharmacol Rev 2015;67(2):462–504.

Bryant CE, Symmons M, Gay NJ. Toll-like receptor signalling through macromolecular protein complexes. Mol Immunol February 2015;63(2):162–5.

De Nardo D. Toll-like receptors: activation, signalling and transcriptional modulation. Cytokine August 2015;74(2):181–9.

Ding J, Wang K, Liu W, She Y, Sun Q, Shi J, et al. Pore-forming activity and structural autoinhibition of the gasdermin family. Nature June 8, 2016;535(7610):111–6.

Eckert JK, Kim YJ, Kim JI, Gürtler K, Oh D-Y, Sur S, et al. The crystal structure of lipopolysaccharide binding protein reveals the location of a frequent mutation that impairs innate immunity. Immunity October 2013;39(4):647–60.

Erridge C, Bennett-Guerrero E, Poxton IR. Structure and function of lipopolysaccharides. Microbes Infect July 2002;4(8):837–51.

Gay NJ, Gangloff M. Structure and function of Toll receptors and their ligands. Annu Rev Biochem 2007;76:141–65.

Gay NJ, Symmons MF, Gangloff M, Bryant CE. Assembly and localization of Toll-like receptor signalling complexes. Nat Rev Immunol 2014;14(8):546–58.

He W, Wan H, Hu L, Chen P, Wang X, Huang Z, et al. Gasdermin D is an executor of pyroptosis and required for interleukin-1β secretion. Cell Res December 2015;25(12):1285–98.

Jang T, Park HH. Crystal structure of TIR domain of TLR6 reveals novel dimeric interface of TIR–TIR interaction for toll-like receptor signaling pathway. J Mol Biol September 2014;426(19):3305–13.

Kawai T, Akira S. The role of pattern-recognition receptors in innate immunity: update on Toll-like receptors. Nat Immunol May 2010;11(5):373–84. Nature Publishing Group.

Kayagaki N, Stowe IB, Lee BL, O'Rourke K, Anderson K, Warming S, et al. Caspase-11 cleaves gasdermin D for non-canonical inflammasome signalling. Nature October 29, 2015;526(7575):666–71.

Kelley SL, Lukk T, Nair SK, Tapping RI. The crystal structure of human soluble CD14 reveals a bent solenoid with a hydrophobic amino-terminal pocket. J Immunol February 1, 2013;190(3):1304–11.

Kim HM, Park BS, Kim JI, Kim SE, Lee J, Oh SC, et al. Crystal structure of the TLR4-MD-2 complex with bound endotoxin antagonist eritoran. Cell 2007;130(5):906–17.

Kim JI, Lee CJ, Jin MS, Lee CH, Paik SG, Lee H, et al. Crystal structure of CD14 and its implications for lipopolysaccharide signaling. J Biol Chem 2005;280(12):11347–51.

Lee CC, Avalos AM, Ploegh HL. Accessory molecules for Toll-like receptors and their function. Nat Rev Immunol 2012;12(3):168–79.

Nyman T, Stenmark P, Flodin S, Johansson I, Hammarström M, Nordlund P. The crystal structure of the human toll-like receptor 10 cytoplasmic domain reveals a putative signaling dimer. J Biol Chem May 2, 2008;283(18):11861–5.

Ohto U, Fukase K, Miyake K, Satow Y. Crystal structures of human MD-2 and its complex with antiendotoxic lipid IVa. Science 2007;316(5831):1632–4.

O'Neill LAJ, Bowie AG. The family of five: TIR-domain-containing adaptors in Toll-like receptor signalling. Nat Rev Immunol May 2007;7(5):353–64.

Park BS, Song DH, Kim HM, Choi B-S, Lee H, Lee J-O. The structural basis of lipopolysaccharide recognition by the TLR4-MD-2 complex. Nature April 30, 2009;458(7242):1191–5.

Poltorak A, He X, Smirnova I, Liu MY, Van Huffel C, Du X, et al. Defective LPS signaling in C3H/HeJ and C57BL/10ScCr mice: mutations in Tlr4 gene. Science December 11, 1998;282(5396):2085–8.

Raetz CR, Whitfield C. Lipopolysaccharide endotoxins. Annu Rev Biochem 2002;71:635–700.

Schumann RR, Leong SR, Flaggs GW, Gray PW, Wright SD, Mathison JC, et al. Structure and function of lipopolysaccharide binding protein. Science September 21, 1990;249(4975):1429–31.

Shi J, Zhao Y, Wang K, Shi X, Wang Y, Huang H, et al. Cleavage of GSDMD by inflammatory caspases determines pyroptotic cell death. Nature October 29, 2015;526(7575):660–5.

Song DH, Lee JO. Sensing of microbial molecular patterns by Toll-like receptors. Immunol Rev 2012;250(1):216–29.

Stowe I, Lee B, Kayagaki N. Caspase-11: arming the guards against bacterial infection. Immunol Rev May 2015;265(1):75–84.

Vanaja SK, Russo AJ, Behl B, Banerjee I, Yankova M, Deshmukh SD, et al. Bacterial outer membrane vesicles mediate cytosolic localization of LPS and caspase-11 activation. Cell May 2016;165(5):1106–19.

Yang J, Zhao Y, Shao F. Non-canonical activation of inflammatory caspases by cytosolic LPS in innate immunity. Curr Opin Immunol 2015;32:78–83. Elsevier Ltd.

Zhao Y, Shao F. Diverse mechanisms for inflammasome sensing of cytosolic bacteria and bacterial virulence. Curr Opin Microbiol February 2016;29:37–42.

Section 4.2

Broz P, Dixit VM. Inflammasomes: mechanism of assembly, regulation and signalling. Nat Rev Immunol June 13, 2016;16(7):407–20.

Chavarría-Smith J, Vance RE. The NLRP1 inflammasomes. Immunol Rev May 2015;265(1):22–34.

Davis BK, Wen H, Ting JP-Y. The inflammasome NLRs in immunity, inflammation, and associated diseases. Annu Rev Immunol April 23, 2011;29:707–35.

Faustin B, Lartigue L, Bruey J, Luciano F, Sergienko E, Bailly-Maitre B, et al. Reconstituted NALP1 inflammasome reveals two-step mechanism of caspase-1 activation. Mol Cell March 9, 2007;25(5):713–24.

Hauenstein AV, Zhang L, Wu H. The hierarchical structural architecture of inflammasomes, supramolecular inflammatory machines. Curr Opin Struct Biol 2015;31:75–83. Elsevier Ltd.

Jin T, Perry A, Jiang J, Smith P, Curry JA, Unterholzner L, et al. Structures of the HIN domain:DNA complexes reveal ligand binding and activation mechanisms of the AIM2 inflammasome and IFI16 receptor. Immunity April 20, 2012;36(4):561–71. Elsevier Inc.

Kagan JC, Magupalli VG, Wu H. SMOCs: supramolecular organizing centres that control innate immunity. Nat Rev Immunol October 31, 2014;14(12):821–6. Nature Publishing Group.

Kersse K, Verspurten J, Vanden Berghe T, Vandenabeele P. The death-fold superfamily of homotypic interaction motifs. Trends Biochem Sci October 26, 2011;36(10):541–52. Elsevier Ltd.

Lamkanfi M, Dixit VM. Mechanisms and functions of inflammasomes. Cell May 22, 2014;157(5):1013–22. Elsevier Inc.

Latz E, Xiao TS, Stutz A. Activation and regulation of the inflammasomes. Nat Rev Immunol May 24, 2013;13(6):397–411.

Lawlor KE, Vince JE. Ambiguities in NLRP3 inflammasome regulation: is there a role for mitochondria? Biochim Biophys Acta April 2014;1840(4):1433–40.

Le HT, Harton JA. Pyrin- and CARD-only proteins as regulators of NLR functions. Front Immunol January 2013;4(September):275.

Lu A, Magupalli VG, Ruan J, Yin Q, Atianand MK, Vos MR, et al. Unified polymerization mechanism for the assembly of ASC-dependent inflammasomes. Cell March 13, 2014;156(6):1193–206.

Lu A, Wu H. Structural mechanisms of inflammasome assembly. FEBS J October 29, 2014;5:1–10.

Lu A, Li Y, Schmidt FI, Yin Q, Chen S, Fu T-M, et al. Molecular basis of caspase-1 polymerization and its inhibition by a new capping mechanism. Nat Struct Mol Biol May 2016;23(5):416–25.

Man SM, Hopkins LJ, Nugent E, Cox S, Glück IM, Tourlomousis P, et al. Inflammasome activation causes dual recruitment of NLRC4 and NLRP3 to the same macromolecular complex. Proc Natl Acad Sci USA May 20, 2014;111(20):7403–8.

Martinon F, Burns K, Tschopp J. The inflammasome: a molecular platform triggering activation of inflammatory caspases and processing of proIL-beta. Mol Cell August 2002;10(2):417–26.

Monie TP. NLR activation takes a direct route. Trends Biochem Sci March 2013;38(3):131–9. Elsevier Ltd.

Muñoz-Planillo R, Kuffa P, Martínez-Colón G, Smith BL, Rajendiran TM, Núñez G. K+ efflux is the common trigger of NLRP3 inflammasome activation by bacterial toxins and particulate matter. Immunity June 27, 2013;38(6):1142–53.

Qin H, Srinivasula SM, Wu G, Fernandes-Alnemri T, Alnemri ES, Shi Y. Structural basis of procaspase-9 recruitment by the apoptotic protease-activating factor 1. Nature June 10, 1999;399(6736):549–57.

Schroder K, Zhou R, Tschopp J. The NLRP3 inflammasome: a sensor for metabolic danger? Science January 15, 2010;327(5963):296–300.

Sharma D, Kanneganti T-D. The cell biology of inflammasomes: mechanisms of inflammasome activation and regulation. J Cell Biol June 20, 2016;213(6):617–29.

Vance RE. The NAIP/NLRC4 inflammasomes. Curr Opin Immunol 2015;32:84–9. Elsevier Ltd.

Wang Y, Yang C, Mao K, Chen S, Meng G, Sun B. Cellular localization of NLRP3 inflammasome. Protein Cell April 23, 2013;4(3):1–7.

Section 4.3

Andersen-Nissen E, Smith KD, Strobe KL, Barrett SLR, Cookson BT, Logan SM, et al. Evasion of Toll-like receptor 5 by flagellated bacteria. Proc Natl Acad Sci USA June 28, 2005;102(26):9247–52.

Andersen-Nissen E, Smith KD, Bonneau R, Strong RK, Aderem A. A conserved surface on Toll-like receptor 5 recognizes bacterial flagellin. J Exp Med February 19, 2007;204(2):393–403.

de Jong HK, Parry CM, van der Poll T, Wiersinga WJ. Host–pathogen interaction in invasive salmonellosis. PLoS Pathog October 4, 2012;8(10):e1002933. Chitnis CE, editor.

Diebolder CA, Halff EF, Koster AJ, Huizinga EG, Koning RI. Cryoelectron tomography of the NAIP5/NLRC4 inflammasome: implications for NLR activation. Structure December 1, 2015;23(12):2349–57.

Dietrich N, Lienenklaus S, Weiss S, Gekara NO. Murine toll-like receptor 2 activation induces type I interferon responses from endolysosomal compartments. PLoS One January 2010;5(4):e10250.

Dougan G, John V, Palmer S, Mastroeni P. Immunity to salmonellosis. Immunol Rev March 2011;240(1):196–210.

Fabrega A, Vila J. *Salmonella enterica* serovar Typhimurium skills to succeed in the host: virulence and regulation. Clin Microbiol Rev April 1, 2013;26(2):308–41.

Halff EF, Diebolder CA, Versteeg M, Schouten A, Brondijk THC, Huizinga EG. Formation and structure of a NAIP5-NLRC4 inflammasome induced by direct interactions with conserved N- and C-terminal regions of flagellin. J Biol Chem November 9, 2012;287(46):38460–72.

Hayashi F, Smith KD, Ozinsky A, Hawn TR, Yi EC, Goodlett DR, et al. The innate immune response to bacterial flagellin is mediated by Toll-like receptor 5. Nature May 26, 2001;410(6832):1099–103.

Hu Z, Zhou Q, Zhang C, Fan S, Cheng W, Zhao Y, et al. Structural and biochemical basis for induced self-propagation of NLRC4. Science October 23, 2015;350(6259):399–404.

Hurley D, McCusker MP, Fanning S, Martins M. Salmonella-host interactions – modulation of the host innate immune system. Front Immunol October 7, 2014;5:481.

Jin MS, Kim SE, Heo JY, Lee ME, Kim HM, Paik S-G, et al. Crystal structure of the TLR1-TLR2 heterodimer induced by binding of a tri-acylated lipopeptide. Cell September 21, 2007;130(6):1071–82.

Kang JY, Nan X, Jin MS, Youn SJ, Ryu YH, Mah S, et al. Recognition of lipopeptide patterns by Toll-like receptor 2-Toll-like receptor 6 heterodimer. Immunity 2009;31(6):873–84.

Kofoed EM, Vance RE. Innate immune recognition of bacterial ligands by NAIPs determines inflammasome specificity. Nature September 29, 2011;477(7366):592–5. Nature Publishing Group.

Lu J, Sun PD. The structure of the TLR5-flagellin complex: a new mode of pathogen detection, conserved receptor dimerization for signaling. Sci Signal May 8, 2012;5(223):pe11.

Lightfield KL, Persson J, Brubaker SW, Witte CE, von Moltke J, Dunipace EA, et al. Critical function for Naip5 in inflammasome activation by a conserved carboxy-terminal domain of flagellin. Nat Immunol October 2008;9(10):1171–8.

Miao EA, Mao DP, Yudkovsky N, Bonneau R, Lorang CG, Warren SE, et al. Innate immune detection of the type III secretion apparatus through the NLRC4 inflammasome. Proc Natl Acad Sci USA February 16, 2010;107(7):3076–80.

McSorley SJ. Immunity to intestinal pathogens: lessons learned from *Salmonella*. Immunol Rev July 2014;260(1):168–82.

Nilsen NJ, Vladimer GI, Stenvik J, Orning MPA, Zeid-Kilani MV, Bugge M, et al. A role for the adaptor proteins TRAM and TRIF in toll-like receptor 2 signaling. J Biol Chem February 6, 2015;290(6):3209–22.

Santos RL. Pathobiology of *Salmonella*, intestinal microbiota, and the host innate immune response. Front Immunol May 26, 2014;5.

Smith KD, Andersen-Nissen E, Hayashi F, Strobe K, Bergman MA, Barrett SLR, et al. Toll-like receptor 5 recognizes a conserved site on flagellin required for protofilament formation and bacterial motility. Nat Immunol December 2003;4(12):1247–53.

Stack J, Doyle SL, Connolly DJ, Reinert LS, O'Keeffe KM, McLoughlin RM, et al. TRAM is required for TLR2 endosomal signaling to type I IFN induction. J Immunol December 15, 2014;193(12):6090–102.

Tenthorey JL, Kofoed EM, Daugherty MD, Malik HS, Vance RE. Molecular basis for specific recognition of bacterial ligands by NAIP/NLRC4 inflammasomes. Mol Cell April 10, 2014;54(1):17–29. Elsevier Inc.

von Moltke J, Ayres JS, Kofoed EM, Chavarría-Smith J, Vance RE. Recognition of bacteria by inflammasomes. Annu Rev Immunol 2012;31:73–106.

Yoon SI, Kurnasov O, Natarajan V, Hong M, Gudkov AV, Osterman AL, et al. Structural basis of TLR5-flagellin recognition and signaling. Science 2012;335(6070):859–64.

Section 4.4

Allen IC, Scull MA, Moore CB, Holl EK, McElvania-TeKippe E, Taxman DJ, et al. The NLRP3 inflammasome mediates in vivo innate immunity to influenza A virus through recognition of viral RNA. Immunity April 17, 2009;30(4):556–65.

Bullough PA, Hughson FM, Skehel JJ, Wiley DC. Structure of influenza haemagglutinin at the pH of membrane fusion. Nature September 1, 1994;371(6492):37–43.

Chen I-Y, Ichinohe T. Response of host inflammasomes to viral infection. Trends Microbiol January 2015;23(1):55–63.

Dash P, Thomas PG. Host detection and the stealthy phenotype in influenza virus infection. Curr Top Microbiol Immunol 2014;386:121–47.

Fleury D, Wharton SA, Skehel JJ, Knossow M, Bizebard T. Antigen distortion allows influenza virus to escape neutralization. Nat Struct Biol February 1998;5(2):119–23.

Goraya MU, Wang S, Munir M, Chen J-L. Induction of innate immunity and its perturbation by influenza viruses. Protein Cell October 24, 2015;6(10):712–21.

Han X, Bushweller JH, Cafiso DS, Tamm LK. Membrane structure and fusion-triggering conformational change of the fusion domain from influenza hemagglutinin. Nat Struct Biol August 2001;8(8):715–20.

Kowalinski E, Lunardi T, McCarthy AA, Louber J, Brunel J, Grigorov B, et al. Structural basis for the activation of innate immune pattern-recognition receptor RIG-I by viral RNA. Cell October 14, 2011;147(2):423–35. Elsevier Inc.

Poeck H, Bscheider M, Gross O, Finger K, Roth S, Rebsamen M, et al. Recognition of RNA virus by RIG-I results in activation of CARD9 and inflammasome signaling for interleukin 1 beta production. Nat Immunol January 2010;11(1):63–9. Nature Publishing Group.

Reikine S, Nguyen JB, Modis Y. Pattern recognition and signaling mechanisms of RIG-I and MDA5. Front Immunol 2014;5:342.

Sauter NK, Hanson JE, Glick GD, Brown JH, Crowther RL, Park SJ, et al. Binding of influenza virus hemagglutinin to analogs of its cell-surface receptor, sialic acid: analysis by proton nuclear magnetic resonance spectroscopy and X-ray crystallography. Biochemistry October 13, 1992;31(40):9609–21.

Weber-Gerlach M, Weber F. Standing on three legs: antiviral activities of RIG-I against influenza viruses. Curr Opin Immunol October 2016;42:71–5.

Wu B, Peisley A, Tetrault D, Li Z, Egelman EH, Magor KE, et al. Molecular imprinting as a signal-activation mechanism of the viral RNA sensor RIG-I. Mol Cell July 2014;55(4):511–23. Elsevier Inc.

Yoneyama M, Onomoto K, Jogi M, Akaboshi T, Fujita T. Viral RNA detection by RIG-I-like receptors. Curr Opin Immunol February 2015;32:48–53.

Section 5

Connecting the Innate and Adaptive Immune Responses

The innate and adaptive immune systems have often historically been viewed as distinct and discrete entities. The absence of an adaptive immune system in invertebrates makes it clear that the innate immune system is able to function independently and is not reliant on the adaptive system to be able to provide an immediate and protective response. Of course the presence of a functional adaptive immune response, while being an obvious advantage in terms of the survival of an individual, does in fact influence the potency and the nature of the innate response. For example, the pattern of cytokine secretion from the T-cell population plays an important role in the global nature of the innate and adaptive responses, with Th1- and Th2-dominant profiles creating proinflammatory and antiinflammatory environments, respectively.

In this section, I will provide different examples to highlight the interplay and connectivity between the innate and the adaptive arms of the immune system. It is not supposed to be an extensive consideration of the minutia of the mechanistic basis of these interactions, but rather a taste of some of the major interactions that occur and their immunological and pathological significance. I will briefly discuss the transcriptional regulation of major histocompatibility complex (MHC) class I and II genes, the interaction between complement and the adaptive immune response, the importance of the dendritic cell as the interface between the innate and adaptive responses, the role of autophagy in the development of B and T cells, and the importance of adjuvant recognition by pattern recognition receptors (PRRs) in the generation of a protective adaptive response following vaccination.

5.1 THE TRANSCRIPTIONAL REGULATION OF MHC CLASS I AND II GENES

The expression of MHC class I and II genes are absolutely crucial to the functionality of the adaptive immune response. MHC, which are also referred to as human leukocyte antigen (HLA) in humans, are expressed on the surface of cells, particularly antigen-presenting cells and lymphocytes. Their role is to enable the specific recognition of peptide fragments within the adaptive immune response. They are particularly important in determining the nature of

The Innate Immune System. http://dx.doi.org/10.1016/B978-0-12-804464-3.00005-3

171

the interaction between T cells, B cells, and antigen-presenting cells and consequently underpin the whole premise of the antigen-specific adaptive immune response.

Almost all cell types express MHC class I, and as we saw in Section 2 the absence of MHC class I on the cell surface can act as a stimulatory signal for the activation of natural killer (NK) cells. In contrast, MHC class II shows a more selective pattern of cellular expression, being located predominantly on antigen-presenting cells. Exposure to proinflammatory cytokines, especially IFNγ, can induce the expression of MHC class II on a more diverse range of cells including, endothelial cells, epithelial cells, and fibroblasts. MHC class I presents antigens derived from inside the cell, such as might result from viral infection. In contrast the MHC class II presentation pathway is used to present extracellular antigens, often of exogenous origin taken up through phagocytosis (Fig. 5.1). The presentation pathways do not discriminate between self and nonself-derived peptides.

The transcriptional regulation of both MHC class I and II, along with those genes that provide accompanying functional roles in peptide processing and presentation, is an essential immune process. It is controlled by two members of the NLR family: NLRC5 and CIITA, which regulate MHC class I and class II gene expression, respectively. Despite minimal sequence identity, CIITA and NLRC5 are phylogenetically close to one another within the NLR family. Unlike other NLR proteins, both CIITA and NLRC5 are found in the cytoplasm and the nucleus.

5.1.1 NLRC5 and the Transcription of MHC Class I Genes

NLRC5 is a member of the NLRC subfamily of NLR proteins. Although NLRC5 possesses an N-terminal CARD, the 3-dimensional fold of this domain deviates slightly from that traditionally observed for CARDs. This might be because of the role of NLRC5 in MHC class I gene expression. NLRC5 is mainly expressed in hematopoietic cells and its levels of expression are increased in response to stimulation with interferons. The ability of NLRC5 to regulate MHC class I gene expression appears to result from its interactions with a multiprotein complex formed from a number of different DNA-binding proteins and transcription factors, which is known as the enhanceosome (Fig. 5.2). The extent of MHC class I expression can be directly correlated to the degree of expression of NLRC5. Genetic depletion of NLRC5 results in a significant reduction in the expression of MHC class I on the surface of cells, a defect that is seen most strongly in immune cells, especially T cells and NK cells.

In addition to its role as a transactivator of MHC class I genes, NLRC5 has also been suggested to play a role in the response to viral infection. However, this aspect of the function of NLRC5 requires further work as different studies report conflicting roles in which NLRC5 acts to suppress, enhance, or has no impact upon, the antiviral response.

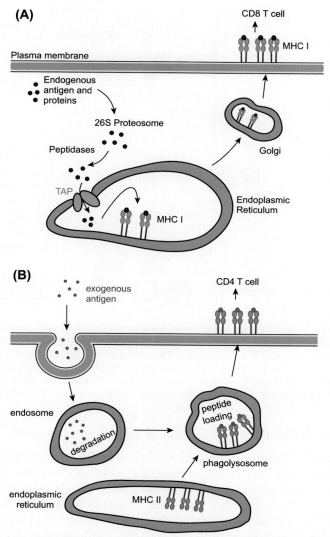

FIGURE 5.1 The presentation of antigenic peptide on major histocompatibility complex (MHC) class I and class II. (A) Native proteins and endogenous antigens in the cytoplasm are targeted for degradation at the 26S proteosome. Digested proteins are further degraded by the action of peptidases leading to the creation of small peptide sequences that are imported via TAP (transporter associated with antigen processing) into the endoplasmic reticulum. Here they are loaded onto MHC class I molecules and then sent to the plasma membrane via the golgi and the secretory pathway. Once at the cell surface, the MHC class I:peptide complex is able to interact with CD8 positive T cells. (B) Exogenous antigens are internalized via endocytic and phagocytic pathways. Proteins are broken down by the action of proteases following formation of a phagolysosome. The peptide fragments are loaded onto MHC class II molecules that are sent to the phagolysosome and then the complex is moved to the plasma membrane from where it can interface with CD4 positive T cells.

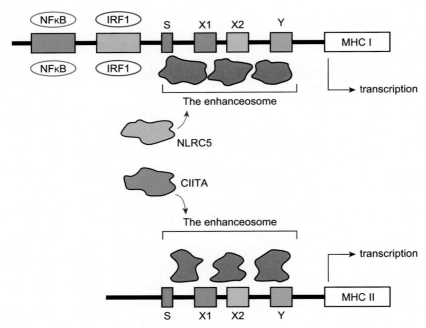

FIGURE 5.2 **A simplified schematic of the promoter regions of major histocompatibility complex (MHC) class I and class II genes.** The promoter regions of MHC class I genes (top) and MHC class II genes (bottom) are quite similar. They contain specific DNA sequences (S, X1, X2 Y) that are recognized by a multiprotein complex known as the enhanceosome. The enhanceosome itself contains a range of proteins including transcription factors such as CREB, NF-Y, and various RX proteins. CIITA, and most probably NLRC5 as well, interact with the enhanceosome to modulate the transcriptional activity of the MHC genes.

5.1.2 CIITA and the Transcription of MHC Class II Genes

Unlike NLRC5, which may possibly function as a PRR, although this require further verification, CIITA does not function as a PRR. CIITA is the sole member of the NLRA subfamily of NLR proteins because of its possession of an N-terminal acidic, or activation, domain that is immediately followed by a series of amino acids rich in serine, threonine, and proline residues. Four different isoforms of CIITA exist, each under the control of a different promoter. Isoform 4 is highly upregulated by IFNγ and isoform 3 is most commonly expressed in plasmacytoid dendritic cells, activated T cells, and B cells, whereas isoform 1 is the dominant isoform in conventional dendritic cells.

CIITA acts as a master regulator of MHC class II gene expression at both the constitutive and the inducible levels. In the absence of CIITA expression, MHC class II expression does not occur. Therefore, cells with constitutive MHC II expression, i.e., APCs, also have constitutive expression of CIITA. CIITA is also responsible for controlling the expression of wide range of accessory proteins that are involved in the correct presentation of peptides via MHC class II. The control that CIITA exerts over MHC II gene expression is not mediated through a direct interaction with the DNA in the MHC II promoter region. Instead, and just like NLRC5, CIITA utilizes the enhanceosome, which contacts the DNA. CIITA then interacts with the enhanceosome and influences the recruitment of histone-modifying enzymes and the general transcription factors required to initiate gene expression (Fig. 5.2).

5.2 COMPLEMENT AND THE ADAPTIVE IMMUNE RESPONSE

We have already seen in Section 3.4.3 that the complement system performs a range of vital innate immune roles. These include the innate recognition (opsonization) and clearance (lysis or stimulated phagocytosis) of pathogens, immune complexes, and dead or dying cells; the production of chemoattractants that recruit immune cells; and the stimulation of proinflammatory cytokine production. However, these are not the only functional roles of complement in the immune defense network and its importance is not limited to the innate response. The complement system also interfaces with the adaptive immune response and influences both B- and T-cell functionality. In fact the importance of complement in shaping and contributing to the adaptive response has become apparent as our understanding of the integrated nature of the immune response has developed. The complement system plays a major role in determining the direction and outcome of both the innate and the adaptive immune responses.

5.2.1 Complement and the Function of B Cells

The fact that B cells express complement receptors—primarily CR2, but also to lesser extent CR1—provides an immediate indication that B-cell function may be influenced by the action or activity of complement. This view is supported by the fact that animal models of complement deficiencies, or in which specific complement components, such as C3, are depleted, can show impaired humoral immunity (i.e., B-cell—driven antibody responses).

The complement molecules are able to bind to foreign material and pathogens throughout the circulation. As part of this process, complement also serves to localize these antigenic compounds into areas in which B- and T-cell lymphocytes accumulate and are activated. The engagement of CR2 serves a range of beneficial functions for the B cell. For example, it stimulates an increase in the surface expression of the B-cell receptor. This is helpful for the generation of both effector and memory B cells within germinal centers during interaction with follicular dendritic cells. Consistent with this a reduction in the level of circulating C3 is associated with a drop in the level of the humoral antibody-driven response.

The presence of complement also serves to reduce the activation threshold of B cells. Binding of the C3 fragment C3d to CR2 results in the formation of a

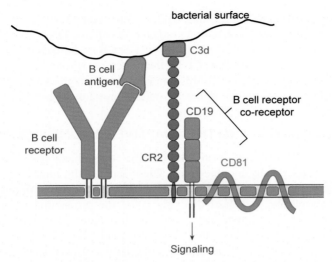

FIGURE 5.3   **The B-cell receptor–coreceptor signaling complex.** The B-cell receptor recognizes antigen on a target surface. The interaction is stabilized through interactions between the
CR2 component of the B-cell receptor–coreceptor with the complement fragment C3d on the target
surface. The coreceptor consists of CR2, CD19, and CD81. CD19 is important for mediating downstream signaling.

coreceptor complex along with CD19 and CD81, which can recognize comple-
ment-opsonized antigens (Fig. 5.3). This process serves to enhance the signal
produced by stimulation of the primary B-cell receptor, but also provides an
adjuvant-like effect and decreases the threshold at which B cells can be activated by up to 10,000-fold. Although in many cases this is advantageous as
it improves the sensitivity with which protective antibodies can be generated
against dangerous pathogens, it can also, however, be problematic. Decreasing
the activation threshold of B cells increases the possibility of generating autoreactive cells that could contribute to the development of autoimmune disorders.
This is believed to be one of the driving mechanisms behind the development of
collagen-induced arthritis.

Complement can also influence presentation of antigens to the B cell by
dendritic cells, which similarly possess complement receptors and are therefore
able to efficiently capture and present complement-labeled antigens. The activation of the CR2 containing coreceptor is also an important part in the overall development of B cells, the activation and instruction of naïve B cells, and
the regulation of B cell death upon low-affinity interactions with antigen. The
regulatory protein C4BP activates the costimulatory receptor CD40 on the surface of B cells. This has the effect of increasing B-cell proliferation, increasing
the surface expression of other important B-cell receptors, such as CD86 and
CD54, and of stimulating the process of isotype switching in relation to the type
of antibody produced. Meanwhile, C4 plays an important role in maintaining

B-cell tolerance and reducing the likelihood of the production of autoantigens targeted against host components, i.e., self-reactive. It has also been suggested that the development of polyclonal B-cell populations, the secretion of proinflammatory TNF and IL-6 by B cells, and B cell migration, are all influenced by the presence of the anaphylatoxins C3a and C5a.

5.2.2 Complement and the T-Cell Response

In addition to influencing B-cell development, stimulation, proliferation, and hence the strength of the protective antibody response, complement also influences T-cell functionality. The mechanisms by which complement and T cells interface with one another are less well understood than for complement and B cells. The inhibition of complement functionality, as a result of the absence of C3, or the impairment of C3 activation, leads to abnormal T-cell function in a variety of infection and allergic settings.

The maintenance of T cells in a resting state is partially dependent on their production of intracellular C3. This protein is then cleaved within the cell and interacts with its receptor, C3aR, on the surface of lysosomes. This process is crucial for continuation of homeostatic functions through its stimulation of basal levels of mTOR signaling and may also happen in other cells as well as T cells. This function cannot be provided by C3a of extracellular origin.

Enhanced complement activity achieved, for example, through the disruption of regulatory functions, has shown that complement is important for the development of a more robust and extensive level of T-cell immunity driven by an enhanced Type I, or Th1, response. This is believed to result from a stimulation of IFNγ and IL-2 secretion, coupled with repression of IL-10, and may potentially be the result of anaphylatoxin-mediated signaling. Once a T cell is activated, it will then express C3aR, in addition to C5aR, on its surface. Engagement of these surface-located receptors by their cognate anaphylatoxin ligands, usually derived from C3 and C5 produced locally by antigen-presenting cells, has a profoundly different effect on the T cell. It stimulates the production of antiapoptotic molecules such as Bcl2, downregulates proapoptotic protein expression, and helps to drive a Th1-based immune response. The absence of this interaction during the activation of T cells causes an increase in the proportion of regulatory T cells produced. In fact, individuals with deficiencies in C3 present with a significant impairment in their ability to initiate a Th1-polarized adaptive immune response. Disruption of C5a-driven signaling leads to a reduction in the production of antigen-specific T cells, inhibits the synergistic interaction between complement and Toll-like receptor (TLR) signaling, and results in a weaker response to a range of infections. T-cell function can also be modulated by proteins such as decay accelerating factor and membrane cofactor protein, which serve to regulate the activation of complement.

5.3 AUTOPHAGY AND THE DEVELOPMENT OF T AND B CELLS

The homeostatic nature of autophagy means that it is bound to be involved in adaptive immune functions, at the very least through maintaining cellular homeostasis in adaptive immune cells. However, there is clear evidence that autophagy makes a variety of different and specific functions to the development, differentiation, and functionality of B and T cells (Fig. 5.4).

Autophagy is important in the maintenance and self-renewal of the hematopoetic stem cells that act as lymphocyte progenitors and continues to play an important role in cellular homeostasis as the cells differentiate. For example, the positive and negative selection, and survival, of thymocytes; the differentiation of Treg and NK cells; the production of metabolites for T-cell proliferation; T-cell survival; and the maintenance of memory T cells, are all believed to be regulated to varying degrees by autophagy. The influence of autophagy on T-cell survival following activation occurs as a result of the destabilization of the immunological synapse that forms during stimulation of the T-cell receptor. Autophagy also directs T cell polarization through an impact on the control of proinflammatory cytokine secretion from other immune cells including macrophages. The survival of mature B cells and plasma cells is also reliant on autophagic functions indicating that the long-term maintenance of a protective antibody–mediated immune response is heavily dependent on the normal functioning of autophagy.

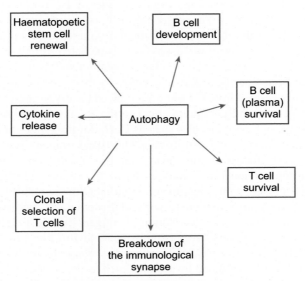

FIGURE 5.4 **The role of autophagy in adaptive immunity.** A schematic representation of some of the roles of autophagy that connect with or influence the adaptive immune response.

Antigen presentation is a crucial part of the training and development of the adaptive immune response and autophagy influences the processes underlying the presentation of antigens on both MHC class I and class II. In some cases, this occurs in conjunction with the activation of autophagy pathways by PRRs such as NOD2.

5.4 THE DENDRITIC CELL IS THE INTERFACE BETWEEN THE INNATE AND THE ADAPTIVE IMMUNE RESPONSE

Dendritic cells are located throughout the body and its tissues and are particularly prominent in surfaces, such as the intestines and the respiratory tract, likely to come into contact with the external environment. They are similarly found at high levels in the lymphatic and circulatory organs that connect to and drain from these surfaces.

The dendritic cell is widely acknowledged as the direct connection between the innate and adaptive arms of the immune response. It is of course not the only link between the two, but it is certainly a crucial, possibly the most important, of all the interfaces present. The importance of dendritic cells in communication between the innate and adaptive arms of the immune response stems predominantly from their interaction with T cells. In fact, dendritic cells are unique, even among antigen-presenting cells, in their phenomenal ability to interact with and stimulate naïve T cells.

Although both dendritic cells and macrophages derive from the same original progenitors and can be grouped together as antigen-presenting cells, it would be inappropriate to classify them as one and the same. Both cell types can, and do, present antigen to naïve T cells. However, this process is much more efficient and functionally important when performed by dendritic cells. In part, this stems from the superior capabilities of the dendritic cell to sample its external environment and therefore more rapidly present a broader range of peptides on its surface, particularly via MHC class II. However, the effector functions of the two cell types also vary. Phagocytosis is a major part of the functional repertoire of macrophages, particularly in relation to the engulfment and destruction of pathogens and the clearance of dead and dying cells. This is not the case for dendritic cells, which could be viewed mostly as an endocytic cell type rather than a phagocytic one. Conventional dendritic cells are also not, unlike macrophages, quite so focused on the production of cytokines. For a long time, it was felt that a dendritic cell was equally able to perform the two key functions, namely antigen presentation and cytokine stimulation. However, it seems more likely now that the dendritic cells can be split into two types: those that perform antigen presentation functions, the presenter dendritic cells, and those that predominantly secrete inflammatory cytokines following PRR-mediated recognition of danger or damage, the detector dendritic cells (Fig. 5.5). An excellent example of this is provided by intestinal dendritic cells in which CD11b$^+$CD103$^+$ cells are more proficient at presenting antigens, and CD11b$^+$CD103$^-$ dendritic cells are

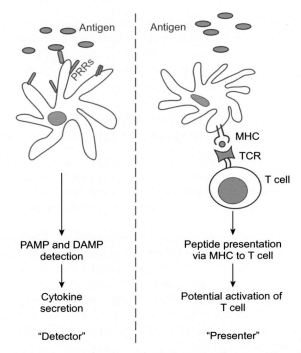

FIGURE 5.5 **Dendritic cells can be viewed as presenters or detectors.** Upon the detection of antigen, there are two basic functions a dendritic cell can perform. It can recognize the antigen as a pathogen-associated molecular pattern or danger/damage-associated molecular pattern via its pattern recognition receptors and subsequently secrete proinflammatory cytokines—a detector. Or it can present peptide fragments of the antigen on major histocompatibility complex to be recognized by T cells, which may then be subsequently activated. These cells are presenters.

particularly proficient at detecting pathogens and stimulating cytokine secretion. To be able to modulate dendritic cell functions for therapeutic use in specific tissue or body locations, it is helpful to know exactly which sorts of cell are present and which function as detectors and as presenters.

We have seen that different types of macrophages exist. These include proinflammatory M1 and antiinflammatory M2 phenotypes, as well as a variety of different tissue-resident macrophages. Different subsets and lineages of dendritic cell also exist. As mentioned in Section 2, there are two main types of dendritic cells—conventional and plasmacytoid. Both types are able to recognize and respond to pathogens and to interact with and activate other immune cells. However, the plasmacytoid dendritic cell is exceptionally efficient at secreting cytokines, particularly type I interferons in response to the detection of viral infection. Meanwhile the conventional dendritic cells are more optimized for the presentation of antigen to T cells and the subsequent activation of these cells.

There is a wide degree of heterogeneity within these two major populations of dendritic cells, which is usually quantifiable through the pattern of receptors expressed on the surface of the dendritic cell. This can be influenced by the location of the dendritic cell, the transcription factors it has expressed, its differentiation history, and by the stimuli it has received. Indeed the complexity of dendritic cell phenotyping has long been problematic, and there is now a move to consider the different types of dendritic cell as being defined by their genetic ontology, rather than by which surface markers they express. Although the major types of dendritic cell show good conservation between humans and mice, it is less clear how accurately the less well-populated and more poorly characterized phenotypes are shared. A very large proportion of our understanding of how dendritic cells function has come from studies using mice and murine dendritic cells. As with many, or maybe any, cross-species studies, this of course means that although the broad functional principles are likely to be conserved, there may well be specific and subtle differences in the way that some murine and human dendritic cells behave and function.

5.4.1 Dendritic Cells and Their Interaction With T Cells

Dendritic cells interact continuously with naïve T cells. They do not require the presence of the pathogen-associated molecular patterns (PAMPs) and danger/damage-associated molecular pattern (DAMPs) that result from danger, infection, and damage, although of course these can serve to increase the rate at which interaction happens and provides a change in the nature of the interaction. Under steady-state (PAMP and DAMP-free) conditions the dendritic cells still present peptides sampled from the external environment, but these will consist predominantly of self-antigens, or inert and innocuous exogenous materials. It is the role of the dendritic cell to ensure that the host becomes tolerant to these stimuli and does not generate a strong, or ideally any, immune response. In contrast, in the presence of PAMPs and DAMPs the dendritic cell becomes a crucial component in the generation of an antigen-specific T cell response and the development of protective immunity.

The interaction between a dendritic cell and a naïve T cell consists of three different signals (Fig. 5.6). Signal 1 results from the antigenic peptide presented on MHC from the dendritic cell interacting with the T-cell receptor complex and either the CD4 or CD8 coreceptor on the T cell. Presentation on MHC class I leads to involvement of the CD8 coreceptor and presentation on MHC class II utilizes the CD4 coreceptor. The second signal is formed from a series of receptor–coreceptor interactions that provide a costimulatory signal to ensure T-cell activation. These interactions include, for example, CD40:CD40 L and CD80 or CD86 with CD28/CTLA4. If there is insufficient costimulation, i.e., a weak signal 2, then the interacting T cell is not activated and instead is instructed to become anergic or to die of apoptosis. Intermediate levels of signal 2 will often result in the generation of memory T cells and therefore contributes to the more rapid adaptive response on subsequent exposure to the same antigen. Some signal 2 interactions are directly inhibitory to T cell activation, for example, the interaction between programmed death

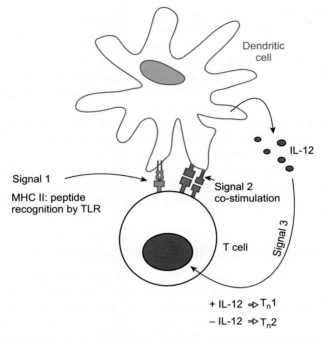

FIGURE 5.6 **The interaction between a dendritic cell and a T cell.** The interaction between a dendritic cell and a T cell consists of three separate signals. Signal 1 is recognition of the major histocompatibility complex (MHC) peptide complex by the TCR. In this figure it is MHC II that would involve CD4 as well as the TCR. If it was MHC I, then the T cells would be CD8 positive. The second signal is the costimulatory signal required for full activation. Costimulation is provided by a number of receptor–coreceptor interactions including CD54:CD11a; CD80:CTLA4; CD86:CTLA4; and CD40:CD40 L. The final signal, signal 3, is provided by the secretion of IL-12 from the dendritic cell. If this occurs, then Th1 responses are favored. If IL-12 secretion does not occur, then Th2 responses are promoted. *TLR*, toll-like receptor.

ligand 1 on the dendritic cell and programmed cell death receptor on the T cell. The various interactions that occur between the dendritic cell and the T cell tend to cluster together in a general area referred to as the immunological synapse. Signal 3 plays a key role in the differentiation of the T cell into a form consistent with either a Th1- or Th2-dominant response. This signal is provided through cytokines secreted by the antigen-presenting dendritic cell and the most important cytokine is IL-12. The presence of IL-12 is a strong driver toward the production of Th1 responses, whereas in its absence, Th2 responses dominate (Fig. 5.6).

The interaction of dendritic cells with T cells is therefore able to dictate the shape and the nature of the primary adaptive immune response both in terms of deciding whether or not a T cell should indeed be activated and in terms of directing the type of T cell produced. This process is influenced by the cytokines secreted by the dendritic cell, which is principally controlled by the detection of, and response to, PAMPs and DAMPs via PRRs. It is this whole process that enables the dendritic cell to provide the functional link between the innate and the adaptive immune responses. Of course, as with many biological systems, the functionality of the dendritic cells is highly complex and they can also directly influence the development of B cells, as well as directing this through the activation of T helper cells.

5.5 ADJUVANTS, PRRs, AND VACCINATION

The process of vaccination can be viewed as one of, if not the, most successful of public health endeavors and has resulted in the saving millions of lives worldwide. At the most basic level, it works around the principle of providing an antigenic stimulus from a pathogen, for example, the tetanus toxoid, in a manner that will not cause clinical disease but does, however, induce a protective adaptive immune response. Classic vaccines that use whole killed or avirulent pathogens or purified toxins in the presence of impurities generally work well in inducing protective immunity. However, on occasion the presence of impurities can induce problematic side effects. There has been a general move toward trying to rationally design vaccines based around known antigenic components and subunits, such as viral surface proteins, produced in a recombinant, highly pure form. However, many of these vaccine candidates have low immunogenicity and fail to induce a sufficient level of protective immunity to make their direct administration viable as a therapeutic intervention. The big driver behind the difference in immunogenicity observed between various types of vaccine candidate is based around the presence, or absence, of molecules that can act as vaccine adjuvants or immune helpers. These are molecules that stimulate PRRs and serve to enhance the immunogenicity of compounds and increase the level of protective antibody and cell-mediated immunity generated. Impure vaccine preparations often contain molecules such as muramyl dipeptide (MDP) and lipopolysaccharide that stimulate the PRRs NOD2 and TLR4, respectively, whereas inactivated or avirulent whole pathogens will possess a whole battery of immunostimulatory PAMPs to act as adjuvants. In contrast, engineered, recombinant, and highly purified molecules almost invariably lack any natural adjuvant capacity and hence need to be administered in conjunction with molecules that provide adjuvant capabilities.

5.5.1 Licensed Adjuvants and the Hunt for New Ones

The mechanism by which adjuvants work clearly has the potential to be dangerous. Any molecule that directly stimulates PRRs may lead to excessive or unintended inflammatory consequences, which, in the most severe cases, could lead to the induction of septic shock or even death. Consequently, there are only a few adjuvants licensed for use in human vaccines. These include aluminum derivatives such as aluminum phosphate and aluminum hydroxide, which are commonly referred to as alum; oil-in-water emulsions such as MF59; and combinations of alum with TLR4 agonists such as mono-phosphorylated lipid A (MPLA). These appear to generally work through stimulation of the NLRP3 inflammasome and/or TLR4 signaling pathways. However, all currently licensed adjuvants suffer from failing to generate a CD8 cytotoxic T-cell response and are therefore poor inducers of cell-mediated Th1 immune responses. This is particularly the case for alum-containing adjuvants. Stimulation of different PRRs can lead to the activation of different signaling profiles that influence whether Th1 or Th2 immune responses dominate. As such, it remains a major goal in vaccine development to generate new and safe adjuvants targeted on certain PRRs. This would then allow the induction of a deliberate profile of cytokines to create a more holistic, realistic, and ultimately protective level of immune response. A similar approach is being taken to target-specific populations of dendritic cells, which could also potentially lead to enhanced memory cell populations in the tissues most likely to encounter a specific pathogen. Currently, clinical trials are occurring to assess the potential of agonists for TLR4, 5, 7, 8, and 9 as vaccine adjuvants.

5.5.2 Adjuvants and PRRs

5.5.2.1 Alum

The mechanism of action by which alum compounds function as vaccine adjuvants remains somewhat controversial. It is clear that their administration increases the uptake and presentation of antigen by dendritic cells and also improves the recruitment of monocytes to the site of inoculation. However, it is currently not entirely clear as exactly which PRRs are involved in helping to drive the adjuvant activity of alum. A number of studies proposed that its effects were mediated through the NLRP3 inflammasome. Other studies have suggested that this may well not be the case. Alum is not proposed to directly activate the NLRP3 inflammasome but may stimulate uric acid production or lead to the release of DNA from dying cells or from damaged mitochondria, which then acts as an immune stimulator. The role of DNA in alum-induced adjuvant activity is gaining in popularity and has been suggested to also function through STING-dependent signaling pathways.

5.5.2.2 Oil-and-Water Emulsions

The manner in which oil-and-water emulsions activate PRRs is somewhat enigmatic as they do not contain molecules that could be viewed as classical PAMPs or DAMPs. However, one such adjuvant MF59 is ASC dependent in its activity. Interestingly, it is not dependent on either NLRP3 or caspase-1 suggesting that although inflammasomes may be involved, these may not be canonical in nature, or at the very least may rely on the activity of other activated caspases, such as caspase-8, rather than caspase-1.

5.5.2.3 Muramyl Dipeptide

MDP activates NOD2, a cytoplasmic PRR to induce a proinflammatory immune response. It is the primary adjuvant component of the widely used experimental adjuvant complete Freunds' adjuvant (CFA). Despite its known capability to function as an adjuvant, the use of MDP has never taken off in human vaccines as it is viewed as being too pyrogenic and therefore having too many potential adverse side effects. To bypass these problems a significant amount of time and effort is being exerted into the creation and testing of MDP analogs and derivatives that retain their NOD2-stimulatory capacity but have reduced potential for the induction of undesirable side effects.

5.5.2.4 Nucleic Acids and Their Analogs

There is a significant level of interest in the use of nucleic acids, their derivatives, and their analogs as vaccine adjuvants. This has focused predominantly on stimulators of the endosomal TLRs and a range of molecules, such as CpG oligonucleotides, are undergoing clinical trials. However, there is an increasing focus on the development of adjuvants that could act as stimulators of the cytoplasmic nucleic acid–sensing PRRs and work through STING-mediated pathways. CpG oligonucleotides are particularly popular candidates for adjuvants in cancer or tumor-specific vaccines as they appear to be particularly effective at creating a cytokine environment conducive to reducing the number of Treg cells in the tumor microenvironment.

It is clear that vaccine adjuvant development remains an area with the potential to rerevolutionize medical therapies and create new vaccine combinations that induce stronger, better lasting levels of immunity, have fewer side effects, require smaller and fewer doses, and can be targeted to produce the most appropriate and relevant type of immune protection to that disease or individual.

REFERENCES AND FURTHER READING

Section 5.1

Devaiah BN, Singer DS. CIITA and its dual roles in MHC gene transcription. Front Immunol 2013;4.

Kobayashi KS, van den Elsen PJ. NLRC5: a key regulator of MHC class I-dependent immune responses. Nat Rev Immunol November 23, 2012;12(12):813–20. Nature Publishing Group.

LeibundGut-Landmann S, Waldburger J-M, Krawczyk M, Otten LA, Suter T, Fontana A, et al. Mini-review: specificity and expression of CIITA, the master regulator of MHC class II genes. Eur J Immunol June 2004;34(6):1513–25.

Lupfer C, Kanneganti T-D. The expanding role of NLRs in antiviral immunity. Immunol Rev September 2013;255(1):13–24.

Neerincx A, Castro W, Guarda G, Kufer TA. NLRC5, at the heart of antigen presentation. Front Immunol 2013;4.

van den Elsen PJ. Expression regulation of major histocompatibility complex class I and class II encoding genes. Front Immunol 2011;2.

Section 5.2

Carroll MC, Isenman DE. Regulation of humoral immunity by complement. Immunity August 24, 2012;37(2):199–207.

Degn SE, Thiel S. Humoral pattern recognition and the complement system. Scand J Immunol August 2013;78(2):181–93.

Dunkelberger JR, Song W-C. Complement and its role in innate and adaptive immune responses. Cell Res January 15, 2010;20(1):34–50.

Kwan W, van der Touw W, Heeger PS. Complement regulation of T cell immunity. Immunol Res December 5, 2012;54(1–3):247–53.

Section 5.3

Botbol Y, Guerrero-Ros I, Macian F. Key roles of autophagy in regulating T-cell function. Eur J Immunol June 2016;46(6):1326–34.

Bronietzki AW, Schuster M, Schmitz I. Autophagy in T-cell development, activation and differentiation. Immunol Cell Biol January 7, 2015;93(1):25–34.

Deretic V. Autophagy as an innate immunity paradigm: expanding the scope and repertoire of pattern recognition receptors. Curr Opin Immunol February 2012;24(1):21–31. Elsevier Ltd.

Deretic V. Autophagy: an emerging immunological paradigm. J Immunol July 1, 2012;189(1):15–20.

Deretic V, Sitoh T, Akira S. Autophagy in infection, inflammation and immunity. Nat Rev Immunol September 25, 2013;13(10):722–37.

Puleston DJ, Simon AK. Autophagy in the immune system. Immunology January 2014;141(1):1–8.

Section 5.4

Benvenuti F. The dendritic cell synapse: a life dedicated to T cell activation. Front Immunol March 7, 2016;7.

Hammad H, Lambrecht BN. Dendritic cells and epithelial cells: linking innate and adaptive immunity in asthma. Nat Rev Immunol March 2008;8(3):193–204.

Iwasaki A, Medzhitov R. Regulation of adaptive immunity by the innate immune system. Science January 15, 2010;327(5963):291–5.

Iwasaki A, Medzhitov R. Control of adaptive immunity by the innate immune system. Nat Immunol March 19, 2015;16(4):343–53.

Lewis KL, Reizis B. Dendritic cells: arbiters of immunity and immunological tolerance. Cold Spring Harb Perspect Biol August 1, 2012;4(8):a007401.

Lipscomb MF, Masten BJ. Dendritic cells: immune regulators in health and disease. Physiol Rev January 1, 2002;82(1):97–130.

O'Keeffe M, Mok WH, Radford KJ. Human dendritic cell subsets and function in health and disease. Cell Mol Life Sci November 5, 2015;72(22):4309–25.

Reizis B, Bunin A, Ghosh HS, Lewis KL, Sisirak V. Plasmacytoid dendritic cells: recent progress and open questions. Annu Rev Immunol 2011;29:163–83.

Williams A, Flavell RA, Eisenbarth SC. The role of NOD-like receptors in shaping adaptive immunity. Curr Opin Immunol February 2010;22(1):34–40.

Section 5.5

Alter G, Sekaly RP. Beyond adjuvants: antagonizing inflammation to enhance vaccine immunity. Vaccine June 8, 2015;33(Suppl. 2):B55–9.

Coffman RL, Sher A, Seder Ra. Vaccine adjuvants: putting innate immunity to work. Immunity October 29, 2010;33(4):492–503. Elsevier Inc.

Liu D, Rhebergen AM, Eisenbarth SC. Licensing adaptive immunity by NOD-like receptors. Front Immunol 2013;4.

Maisonneuve C, Bertholet S, Philpott DJ, De Gregorio E. Unleashing the potential of NOD- and Toll-like agonists as vaccine adjuvants. Proc Natl Acad Sci USA August 26, 2014;111(34):12294–9.

Oleszycka E, Lavelle EC. Immunomodulatory properties of the vaccine adjuvant alum. Curr Opin Immunol June 2014;28:1–5.

Shirota H, Tross D, Klinman D. CpG oligonucleotides as cancer vaccine adjuvants. Vaccines May 8, 2015;3(2):390–407.

Spreafico R, Ricciardi-Castagnoli P, Mortellaro A. The controversial relationship between NLRP3, alum, danger signals and the next-generation adjuvants. Eur J Immunol March 2010;40(3):638–42.

Suresh R, Mosser DM. Pattern recognition receptors in innate immunity, host defense, and immunopathology. AJP Adv Physiol Educ December 1, 2013;37(4):284–91.

Section 6

The Innate Immune System in Health and Disease

Somewhat unsurprisingly, one can connect the innate immune system to almost all, if not indeed all, types of disease. The ability of the innate immune system to not only detect and respond to exogenous dangers and threats, but also to recognize endogenously derived danger signals shows that it plays a crucial role in the maintenance of homeostasis and the resolution of damage. Earlier sections of this book have already highlighted the myriad of roles and functions that the innate immune system possesses and the main ways in which it exerts an impact on the host. Section 4, in particular, focuses on the specific responses to bacterial and viral threat and reiterates the connectivity and cross talk present between the different arms of the innate response. While in Section 5 the integral importance of the innate immune system in relation to the appropriate activation of both natural adaptive immunity and vaccine-induced immunity is highlighted. In this section, I move on to discuss the role of the innate immune response in the induction and the continuation of major noninfectious public health threats— most notably, cardiovascular disease, rheumatoid arthritis (RA), autoinflammatory syndromes, and inflammatory bowel disease (IBD). In each of these case studies I will provide an overview of the functional mechanisms by which innate immunity contributes to disease and relate these to longer-term prospects for disease management or treatment. A more in-depth consideration of each condition can be obtained by considering the References and Further Reading at the end of the section.

6.1 INFLAMMATION AND ATHEROSCLEROSIS

Atherosclerosis is the underlying cause of strokes and myocardial infarction (heart attack). It provides a clear example of a long-term chronic inflammatory condition that carries a high level of morbidity and mortality. Atherosclerosis results from extended and continuous damage to the vascular endothelium, oxidative stress, and the deposition of lipids. Over the years, there have been a number of suggestions that infection is an important contributor to the maintenance of the inflammatory state associated with atherosclerosis. However, as our understanding of inflammatory mechanisms and stimuli has developed, it has become apparent that there are plenty of endogenous and

The Innate Immune System. http://dx.doi.org/10.1016/B978-0-12-804464-3.00006-5

disease-associated compounds that function as chronic stimulants of inflammation. These include oxidized lipoproteins such as oxLDL and cholesterol crystals.

Macrophages play a major role in the development and pathogenesis of atherosclerosis. The role of the macrophage in atherosclerosis begins with the very first endothelial injury events. Circulating LDL accumulates at the site of injury. Monocytes that are recruited to the site of damage differentiate into macrophages following stimulation with M-CSF. Much of the deposited LDL is converted to oxLDL through the action of ROS and enzymatic cleavage, a proinflammatory molecule that has a high affinity for uptake by macrophages (Fig. 6.1). Consequently the macrophages present at the site of injury begin to phagocytose the oxLDL. OxLDL uptake occurs mainly through interactions with scavenger receptor A (SR-A) and CD36, surface proteins that are in essence functioning as a form of pattern recognition receptor (PRR). Uptake of oxLDL via CD36, which is expressed at high levels on the macrophage surface, results from a high-affinity interaction in which amino acids 155–183 on CD36 play a key role. The binding between CD36 and oxLDL stimulates lipid raft–mediated endocytosis as opposed to the classical caveolin or clathrin-driven pathways. SR-A is also highly expressed on macrophages and the presence of oxLDL and the action of proinflammatory cytokines serve to increase its expression levels further. Consequently there is interest in developing therapeutic approaches that decrease the expression of these receptors and therefore reduce the uptake of oxLDL by macrophages. Natural products such as some polyphenols and circumin are believed to exert some of their health benefits through this sort of effect. Classical preventative treatments such as statins and antihypertensives work by reducing LDL levels and reducing endothelial injury, respectively. While very effective in lessening the development of new plaques, these treatments are limited with respect to the impact they have on atherosclerotic plaques that have already developed.

Once the oxLDL has been internalized by the macrophage, it is then metabolized. This causes the lipids, including cholesterol, to be esterified and either stored for future use or exported from the macrophage into HDL particles. Excess levels of oxLDL can unbalance these metabolic fluxes and efflux processes and lead to an enhancement of lipid accumulation in the macrophages. This can ultimately lead to the accumulation of such high levels of lipid that it nearly fills the cytoplasm of the macrophage and results in the formation of a foam cell. High levels of oxLDL can also lead to incomplete esterification of internalized cholesterol and the subsequent deposition of free cholesterol in a crystalline form on the vessel walls. These crystals can act as a major inflammatory mediator through activation of the NLRP3 inflammasome (Fig. 6.1).

Macrophages are retained in the developing atherosclerotic plaque partly as a result of an increase in the expression of molecules like nectin-1 that inhibit macrophage migration. This helps to contribute to the prolonged

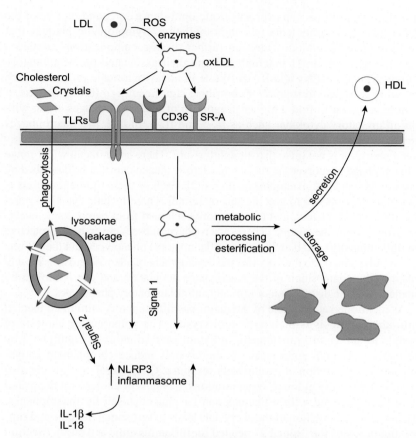

FIGURE 6.1   Uptake of oxidized LDL and cholesterol crystals contribute to the proinflammatory phenotype of macrophages in atherosclerosis. LDL is oxidized by the action of ROS and enzymatic cleavage to generate its oxidized form oxLDL. Scavenger receptors and TLRs on the macrophage surface internalize, or are activated, by oxLDL. The activation of TLRs provides "Signal 1" to prime the NLRP3 inflammasome and will also stimulate a proinflammatory phenotype via cytokine and chemokine secretion and ROS production. The oxLDL is metabolically processed via esterification by the macrophage to be secreted in HDL particles or stored. Excess oxLDL leads to increased storage without processing and the formation of foam cells. The internalization of cholesterol crystals can induce lysosomal damage and rupture and therefore provides "Signal 2" for the NLRP3 inflammasome resulting in IL-1β and IL-18 secretion. TLR activation also serves to stimulate the production of proinflammatory cytokines, chemokines, inflammatory enzymes, and ROS.

inflammatory status. Within the plaque, both proinflammatory (M1) and anti-inflammatory (M2) macrophages are found. The relative proportion of each macrophage phenotype is an important determinant in the potential pathogenesis of a plaque and the progression of disease. Factors influencing progression include narrowing of the blood vessel as the plaque continues to grow, formation of a fibrous cap over a necrotic lipid-dense core, and rupture of the plaque to release fragments into the circulation. Symptomatic plaques that have a higher likelihood of driving further disease complications contain a higher proportion of M1 macrophages and their associated proinflammatory cytokines such as IFNγ and IL-1β. While in nonsymptomatic plaques, which are unlikely to lead to rupture or contribute significantly to further disease, it is more common to find a higher proportion of M2 macrophages along with antiinflammatory cytokines such as IL-3 and IL-4. In fact, M2 macrophages are associated with a reduction in disease progression.

Of course, it is not quite that straightforward. There are in fact a wider range of macrophage phenotypes in the atherosclerotic plaque than can be described by classical M1 and M2 macrophages (Fig. 6.2). Each of these different subsets is created in the response to specific sets of stimuli. These include cytokines, chemokines, growth factors, and heme and iron released from hemorrhagic events occurring within the plaque. These macrophage subsets cover both protective (antiinflammatory) and damaging (proinflammatory) phenotypes and their diversity provides support to the view that the development of atherosclerosis is closely linked to the composition of the macrophage population and can be driven by imbalances in the distribution of pro- and antiinflammatory phenotypes.

As mentioned earlier, one of the major proinflammatory stimuli connected with atherosclerosis is the cholesterol crystal. The potential for cholesterol crystals to act as an immunogenic inflammatory stimulus is highlighted by the fact that at high concentrations the crystals induce complement activation and the generation of an antibody response. Cholesterol crystals are also immunostimulatory at lower concentrations. Crystals of cholesterol deposited on vessel walls and within plaques can be phagocytosed by macrophages. Excessive internalization of these crystals leads to lysosomal damage and rupture and provides the "signal 2" needed for inflammasome activation (Section 4.2). Signal 1, or NLRP3 priming, can be provided by the internalization of oxLDL. As such, cholesterol crystals can stimulate NLRP3 inflammasome activation in a pathogen-free, i.e., sterile manner. The IL-1β subsequently produced from these macrophages as a product of NLRP3 inflammasome activation is proinflammatory and contributes to driving disease. Without question, macrophage-driven innate inflammatory responses are key to the development and the progression of atherosclerosis and its related cardiovascular complications.

6.2 RHEUMATOID ARTHRITIS

RA is already one of the most common chronic inflammatory diseases affecting between 0.5% and 1% of the global population. Worryingly the incidence of RA appears to be increasing. RA predominantly targets the synovial joints, which experience an influx and gradual accumulation of activated inflammatory cells. RA is therefore described as an articular disease, and the musculoskeletal effects of the condition become increasingly debilitating as the disease progresses. In

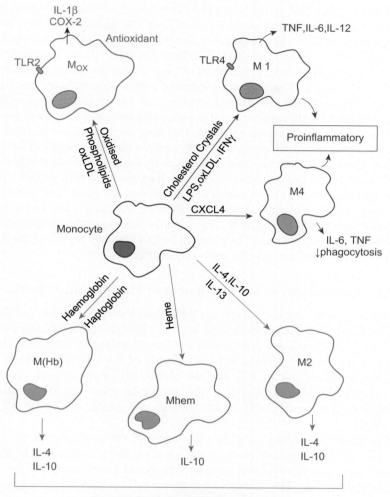

FIGURE 6.2   Schematic representation of the different macrophage phenotypes found in the atherosclerotic plaque. A range of different macrophage phenotypes are found in the atherosclerotic plaque with both proinflammatory and antiinflammatory characteristics. The major stimuli inducing phenotype differentiation are shown as the primary cytokine secretions and functional roles of each phenotype. M1 and M4 are proinflammatory, M2, Mhem and M(Hb) are antiinflammatory, and Mox provides antioxidant functions to limit conversion of LDL to oxLDL. The balance between the numbers of each macrophage phenotype dictates disease progression.

the most severe cases, destruction of the joint may occur. Systemic complications are commonly seen with RA, and these can include, vasculitis, widespread rheumatic nodule deposition, increased risk of cancer, elevated morbidity with cardiovascular disease, and osteoporosis.

The etiology of RA is highly complex, incompletely defined, and involves a variety of genetic and environmental factors. Over 100 separate genes have been connected to an increased risk of developing RA, many of which are involved in key innate (IL-6, TRAF1, IRAK1) and adaptive (CD28, CD40) immune functions. The most common and important of these genetic loci is the human leukocyte antigen (HLA), which is the dominant genetic susceptibility factor for the development of RA. The HLA system encodes for the major histocompatibility complex (MHC) proteins used to present antigenic peptides for recognition by the adaptive immune response. Therefore the importance of HLA in the development and progression of RA suggests that the process of MHC-peptide presentation, binding, and recognition are critical. Consistent with this, RA patients often possess autoantibodies against modified host peptides and IgG. Treatment clears the disease in a small minority of cases, and remission is usually the targeted clinical outcome. However, even this is less commonly achieved than would be desirable. This is partly because of the complexity of the disease and partly because of a current lack of certainty regarding the best cellular and molecular targets for intervention strategies.

6.2.1 The Initiation and Establishment of Rheumatoid Arthritis

It is unclear what exactly precipitates the inflammatory phenotype that ultimately leads to the development of RA. As highlighted earlier, there is a clear genetic component that influences disease susceptibility rather than acting as a causative element. A family history of RA results in a three- to fivefold increased risk of RA, and the heritability of the disease falls in the range of 20–50% depending on the level of seropositivity for autoantibodies—the greater the level of autoantibody the greater the likelihood of heritability.

Environmental factors certainly play a part in the establishment of RA. Positive risk factors include smoking and a low socioeconomic status. In addition a range of microorganisms have been proposed to act as triggers for the initiation of disease. This includes generalized dysregulation of the intestinal microbiome, infection with Epstein–Barr virus, *Proteus mirablis*, or perhaps most convincingly the periodontal pathogen *Porphyromonas gingivalis*.

Regardless of the precise trigger, the earliest events in RA pathogenesis involve activation of innate immune cells, particularly antigen-presenting cells such as dendritic cells and macrophages by both exogenous and endogenous ligands. These cells then serve not only to produce proinflammatory cytokines, but also to activate further immune effector cells including T and B cells. This produces a proinflammatory feedback loop that exacerbates disease. The development of synovitis results from the infiltration of innate immune cells (macrophages, neutrophils, mast cells, natural killer cells, innate lymphoid cells) into the synovial fluid and the subsequent secretion of proinflammatory mediators leading to long-term chronic damage.

6.2.2 The Role of Cytokines in the Pathogenesis of Rheumatoid Arthritis

The pathogenesis of RA is driven by a complex interplay of inflammatory factors and immune cells. The repertoire of cytokines involved is broad and includes TNFα, IL-6, IL-1, interferons, GM-CSF, IL-17, IL-21, IL-23, and IL-12. Of these the proinflammatory cytokines TNFα and IL-6 play a particularly important role. TNFα is often reported to be the pivotal cytokine in RA pathogenesis, and it certainly provides a large repertoire of functions relevant to the progression of disease. These include the activation of multiple cell types including endothelial cells, stromal cells, chondrocytes, leukocytes (including enhancing their migration), and osteoclasts within the synovial environment. Similar effects are also brought about through the action of IL-6. The proinflammatory environment is further enhanced by the secretion of matrix metalloproteinases that degrade the cartilage, causing the release of danger/damage-associated molecular patterns (DAMPs) and leading to continual inflammation and swelling of the synovial membrane and enhancement of the disease. The activation of osteoclasts results from the production of macrophage colony-stimulating factor and RANK ligand and is particularly important for the longer-term pathology because these multinucleated cells are the major cause of bone destruction. T and B cells are also recruited to the synovium where they contribute to the proinflammatory phenotype. This is enhanced by the presence of IL-17, which shares some functionality with both TNFα and IL-6.

6.2.3 Rheumatoid Arthritis, Pattern Recognition Receptors, and Therapy

The importance of proinflammatory cytokines in the pathogenesis of RA shows that PRRs are also an important player in the dynamics of disease progression. In fact Toll-like receptors (TLRs) and nucleotide-binding, leucine-rich repeat–containing receptor (NLRs) have both been associated with a number of arthritis-like conditions in addition to RA, which include psoriatic arthritis, ankylosing spondylitis, and osteoarthritis. In the case of RA the evidence for TLR involvement is strong and patients routinely display raised levels of TLR5 expression on cells in the peripheral circulation, as well as increased expression of TLR2, 3, 4, 7, and 9 in the inflamed joints themselves. Increases in the expression levels of NOD1 and NOD2 have also been reported. In addition, NLRP3 may well play an important role in the contribution to disease progression via the production of IL-1β.

Proinflammatory cytokines and the PRRs that stimulate their production present an obvious therapeutic target for the treatment of RA and other chronic inflammatory conditions. Conventional treatment of RA has involved the use of methotrexate, corticosteroids, and nonsteroidal antiinflammatory drugs. More recently there has been an increase in the use of biologics aimed at inhibiting or neutralizing the cytokine directly. These include anti-TNF and anti-IL-6 receptor antibodies. Clinical trials have suggested that anti-IL-1 treatments also have the potential to improve disease prognosis. Interestingly, positive clinical outcomes upon anti-IL-1 therapy do not necessarily correlate with a similar reduction in the levels of observable inflammation. This reinforces the view that RA pathogenesis is complex and multifactorial. Although the clinical outcomes of biology-based treatments are often improved compared to classical approaches, they do have drawbacks. Up to 30% of patients fail to respond and treatments are much more costly than conventional therapies. This limits the situations they can be used in. Administration is also more invasive and systemic side effects can be seen up on the suppression of TNF, IL-1, and IL-6 responses that may lead to increased susceptibility to infections as a result of immunosuppression. If treatment is stopped, reactivation of disease can be rapid.

A deeper understanding of the processes that lead to the development and progression of RA provides the potential for developing new therapeutic options. Ideally these would work earlier in the disease cascade and address causative elements of the inflammation, rather than relying on neutralizing the effector molecules expressed. As such, there is particular interest in targeting those TLRs and NLRs that show increased expression in the diseased synovium. Of course at the moment, there is only limited understanding of what the long-term impact of the chronic impairment of specific PRR function might be. For example, would a higher incidence of other diseases, or particular infections, be observed? Or, would the activity of other PRR pathways increase to provide functional redundancy and lead to a reestablishment of disease? These are questions that no doubt will be answered in the future.

6.3 AUTOINFLAMMATORY SYNDROMES

The term autoinflammation is generally used to refer to conditions where an inflammatory response occurs as a result of dysfunction or failure of the innate immune system. Classical descriptions of autoinflammatory conditions do not include diseases that are the result of autoreactive B or T cells. Autoinflammatory conditions do not require an infectious stimulus. Early studies of autoinflammatory disorders tended to focus on conditions with a "classical" set of clinical manifestations that included recurrent fever, arthritic or cutaneous involvement, and abdominal pain or discomfort. However, more recently understanding of the molecular mechanisms that underpin autoinflammatory disorders has improved. Consequently the diversity of conditions encompassed by the term has widened, and it is now clear that there are a variety of different mechanisms by which autoinflammatory diseases can be caused. For example, they may result from protein misfolding as occurs with TNF receptor–associated periodic fever syndrome or chronic atypical neutrophilic dermatosis with lipodystrophy and elevated temperature. This last disease leads to increased levels of type I interferon production, a phenotype also seen with Aicardi–Goutières syndrome and has led to a whole host of autoinflammatory disorders being classified as interferonopathies. Autoinflammatory disorders may also result from mutations in proteins, particularly PRRs, which leads to them acquiring an autoactive conformation and hence permits inflammatory signaling even in the absence of stimulatory ligand. An example of this is provided by the disorder Blau syndrome, which is caused by mutations in the central NACHT region of the PRR NOD2 and which appears to disrupt the formation of the autoinhibited conformation of the receptor.

An increase in the levels of type I interferon is one example of how autoinflammatory disorders can manifest themselves. What is more commonly observed, however, is an increased production of the proinflammatory cytokine interleukin-1, particularly interleukin-1β, and it is conditions that lead to enhanced IL-1β production that I shall mainly discuss. We saw in Section 4.2 that a major source of IL-1β is the inflammasome, and consequently, mutations and polymorphisms in proteins that regulate, or drive, the assembly and regulation of the inflammasome have the potential to create an autoactive phenotype analogous to that seen with NOD2 in Blau Syndrome. In these inflammasome-related conditions, the net result is an increase in the production of IL-1β. The family of conditions that are affected by dysregulation of inflammasome-mediated IL-1β production are often referred to as periodic fevers. They include conditions such as familial Mediterranean fever (FMF), the cryopyrin-associated periodic syndromes (CAPS), and macrophage activation syndrome (MAS). Usually, each of these conditions is hereditary, although sporadic cases are not unknown. I will discuss each of these in more detail in the sections that follow.

6.3.1 Familial Mediterranean Fever

FMF is often referred to as the prototypical autoinflammatory disorder and is the most common manifestation of this disease type. It results from activating mutations in the *MEFV* gene, which encodes the inflammasome-forming protein Pyrin. The disease normally presents as brief periods of recurrent fever that are accompanied with painful inflammation in the lungs, abdomen, and the joints. These inflammatory episodes tend to be self-limiting and resolve spontaneously. However, a long-term consequence of the condition can be the development of amyloidosis.

FMF is an inherited disorder and therefore commonly seen in families. It is normally described as an autosomal recessive condition meaning that individuals may act as carriers of the disease if they possess one mutant allele and one wild-type allele. However, the reality may not be that simple. An increasing number of heterozygotic individuals who present with clinical symptoms indistinguishable, albeit slightly milder, from those displayed by homozygotic individuals are being identified. This highlights the genetic complexity of the disease. It may reflect the influence of other genetic factors, environmental variation, or even epigenetic changes. However, a major contributory factor is likely to be the actual mutation itself in the *MEFV* gene. Over 300 distinct mutations have been reported, the majority of which do not lead to clinical disease. Certain changes, such as mutation of the methionine at position 694 in the Pyrin protein, are known to be associated with more severe disease phenotypes. FMF can afflict any genetic background but is especially common in populations of Mediterranean descent.

6.3.2 Cryopyrin-Associated Periodic Syndromes

The CAPS represent a spectrum of diseases that all result from mutations in the inflammasome-forming protein NLRP3. The NLRP3 protein, as well as the gene encoding for it, have had numerous names over the years as a result of different groups of scientists describing and associating particular physiological functions and disease phenotypes with it. These have included "cold auto-inflammatory syndrome 1" and "cryopyrin" in connection with the periodic syndromes. The repertoire of CAPS is broadly characterized through three distinct conditions: Muckle–Wells syndrome (MWS), familial cold autoinflammatory syndrome (FCAS), and neonatal-onset multisystem inflammatory disease (NOMID). NOMID is sometimes called chronic infantile neurologic cutaneous articular syndrome. In humans the mildest of these conditions is FCAS and the most severe is NOMID.

Like FMF the CAPSs result from gain-of-function mutations, although this time in the NLRP3 protein rather than the Pyrin protein. To date, over 170 different mutations in NLRP3 have been associated with CAPS. Some mutations appear to be specific to a single disease. For example, A352V is linked to MWS. Other mutations are connected to more than one type of CAPS— R260W can cause both MWS and FCAS. All of these gain-of-function CAPS mutations result in the overproduction of IL-1β, which is the primary driver of the systemic, the tissue-specific, and the organ-specific inflammation observed with the diseases. Clinically, all forms of the CAPS display periodic and recurrent outbreaks of systemic inflammation that is characterized by rashes on the skin, often triggered by exposure to the cold. The conditions first manifest during early childhood and is associated with inflammation in locations such as the joints, bones, and eyes. The most severe forms of CAPS are often symptomatic at an even earlier age and display a wide range of additional symptoms of varying severity, which can include swelling of the meninges, overgrowth of bones, stunted growth, dysmorphia, and mental retardation.

Even though the physiological cause of FMF and the CAPS is essentially the same—overproduction of IL-1β—the genetics are different. FMF is an autosomal recessive disease, whereas the CAPS are autosomal dominant disorders. Hence, only a single allele needs to be mutated to cause CAPS. This difference most likely results from the fact that the two different proteins that are mutated in the conditions have slightly different functions. Although both Pyrin and NLRP3 form inflammasomes and stimulate IL-1β, the NLRP3 inflammasome is more important and a more potent contributor to cellular levels of IL-1β. In fact it has been suggested that Pyrin may well function as a negative regulator of IL-1β production. Consequently, gain-of-function mutations in NLRP3 have a greater potential, compared with those in Pyrin, for perturbing IL-1β levels. This may be further exacerbated by the pattern of protein expression displayed by Pyrin within white blood cells. Unlike NLRP3, Pyrin is more predominant in granulocytes and only present at low levels in monocytes. This again will reduce the systemic impact of Pyrin mutation, whereas NLRP3, which is widely expressed in monocytes and macrophages, has a much greater scope for influencing systemic IL-1β levels.

6.3.3 Macrophage Activation Syndrome

Rheumatoid diseases, particularly in children, can in rare cases lead to the development of the potentially fatal condition of MAS. More recently, MAS has also been reported in sufferers of periodic inflammatory syndromes and other autoinflammatory conditions. There is no one specific trigger for the activation of MAS, and it may be connected directly to the underlying disease state, be triggered by infection, result from therapeutic changes or interventions, or occur spontaneously. Fairly recently, genetic mutations in the NACHT region of the PRR NLRC4 have been reported to lead to the induction of MAS as a result of compromising the autoinhibited state of the inactive receptor (Fig. 6.3).

The diagnosis of MAS is often hard to make because many of the clinical symptoms, such as high fever, the development of encephalopathy, and dysfunctions in the hepatic and circulatory system, are highly similar to those that occur during sepsis. Indeed, MAS can be an additional complication of sepsis. One of the major effects of MAS is hemophagocytic activity in the bone marrow—the eating of blood cells—and this is a large contributor to the pathogenesis of the condition. The severity of the disease means that rapid diagnosis is essential because otherwise it becomes increasingly difficult to control the excessive production of cytokines that commonly occurs with the disease.

6.3.4 Autoinflammatory Syndromes Can Result From Defects in IL-1 Family Member Antagonists

The previous conditions are all the result of dysregulated IL-1β production. They also show changes in the levels of IL-18, another member of the IL-1

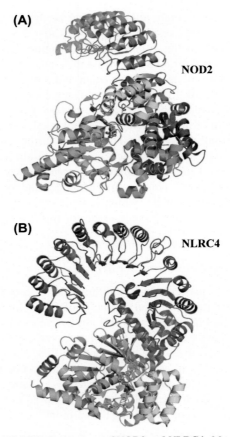

FIGURE 6.3   The autoinhibited structures of NOD2 and NLRC4. Members of the NLR family are believed to exist in an autoinhibited state, which is disrupted by mutations that interfere with ADP binding, protein contacts involved in stabilization of the inhibited conformation, and disrupt chaperone protein binding. The autoinhibited structures of (A) NOD2 and (B) NLRC4 are shown. Both structures were solved in the absence of their N-terminal CARDs. In each case the proteins are colored by domain: nucleotide-binding domain (NBD)—cyan; helical domain 1 (HD1)—yellow; winged helix domain (WHD)—green; helical domain 2 (HD2)—deep red; and leucine-rich repeats (LRRs)—blue. The bound ADP molecule in the Walker A site of the NBD is shown in *stick* representation and colored orange. In addition to the binding of ADP the NLRC4 autoinhibited conformation is stabilized by contacts between the NBD and the LRRs and HD2. The NOD2 conformation is stabilized in particular by interactions between the NBD with the WHD, HD1, and HD2 but especially by contacts between the WHD and HD2.

cytokine family, because of the shared inflammasome-driven mechanism of activation between IL-1β and IL-18. Quite how the balance of IL-1β and IL-18 levels influences the clinical progression of the diseases is, however, not currently clear. IL-1–associated autoinflammatory disorders can also result from genetically induced deficiencies in members of the IL-1 family, which have antagonist functions. A full consideration of all of these conditions goes beyond the scope of this work; however, they can be exemplified by the conditions of deficiency in IL-1 receptor antagonist (DIRA) and deficiency in IL-36 receptor antagonist (DITRA). DIRA results in a severe systemic autoinflammatory disorder that leads to skeletal deformity and may result in lung disease and vasculitis. DITRA, on the other hand, is characterized by generalized pustular psoriasis and does not involve the systemic inflammation observed with DIRA or other conditions that affect IL-1, as opposed to IL-36, signaling pathways.

6.3.5 Treatment of Periodic Inflammatory Disorders

The treatment of periodic inflammatory disorders is focused on suppressing the inflammatory phenotype and the methods used are applicable across the different conditions, albeit with differing levels of efficacy. In most cases the aim is to bring the fever under control, manage the associated pain, and tackle the symptoms relevant to the disease. Immunosuppression and a reduction in inflammation can be achieved by targeting the source of increased inflammatory signaling, by targeting the outputs of the inflammatory cascades activated, or by creating a general immunosuppressive state. Nonsteroidal antiinflammatory drugs, which work by targeting cyclooxygenase and hence disrupt leukotriene and eicosanoid biosynthesis, are commonly used to help control the pain, fever, and early inflammatory response. In addition, antiinflammatory steroids, such as prednisone, are widely used in the early stages of treatment, but they are not generally viewed as a long-term, or indeed an optimal, treatment option. An increasingly common occurrence is the use of antibody-based therapy, such as through the use of anti-IL-1 or anti-TNF biologics. Anti-TNF therapies, such as Etanercept, have proved highly effective in some individuals but appear to exacerbate symptoms in others. On the other hand, anti-IL-1–based treatments are generally much better tolerated and provide better control of the diseases. Short-term treatment is most commonly provided by the administration of the IL-1 receptor antagonist anakinra. Longer-term treatment more often uses Rilonacept or Canakinumab. Canakinumab is a monoclonal antibody that neutralizes IL-1β, whereas Rilonacept is a recombinant protein that provides high-affinity binding for IL-1α, IL-1β, and the IL-1 receptor accessory protein, thereby reducing the biological availability of these effectors. Biologic-based treatments generally produce significant clinical improvement, although they are expensive. However, because of the broad roles of molecules such as TNF and IL-1 in the inflammatory response, they can also induce broader immunosuppressive effects. This has the potential to lead to further complications and may increase the susceptibility of the patient to other conditions or to infection. Research into the development of new specific therapies for these disorders is therefore a priority.

The treatment of FMF commonly involves the administration of the plant extract colchicine, which is from the autumn crocus (*Colchicum autumnale*). The presence of colchicine in the autumn crocus actually serves to make the plant poisonous, and there have been documented fatalities as a result of ingestion of the plant. Colchicine works by binding to alpha and beta tubulin and interfering with microtubule polymerization in cells, which has a number of broadly antiinflammatory effects. This includes a reduction in the production of IL-1β due to inhibition of the NLRP3 inflammasome—for this reason colchicine is also used as a treatment for gout, which is driven by the activation of the NLRP3 inflammasome by uric acid crystals. In FMF the disruption of microtubules by colchicine may well also inhibit Pyrin-driven inflammasome formation and help to compensate for any loss in regulation of the NLRP3 inflammasome. It has also been suggested that it may interfere with the expression of the *MEFV* gene. Further contributions to the antiinflammatory effects of colchicine result from the following conditions: (1) reductions in NFκB expression; (2) a decrease in E-selectin and D-selectin expression on endothelial cells and neutrophils, respectively; (3) inhibition of mast cell degranulation; (4) enhanced TGF-β production; and (5) a decrease in the surface expression of TNF-α receptors on macrophage and epithelial cells.

MAS has a set of treatment options similar to those used in RA. Initial treatment is with high doses of corticosteroids and glucocorticoids. This is sometimes followed with, or performed in parallel with, cyclosporine A and cyclophosphamide treatment to try and limit the activity of lymphocytes. Another common approach is the administration of intravenous immunoglobulin. Anti-TNF treatments have appeared to be quite successful in many cases, but there are some fears that this could in fact trigger MAS in some individuals. Anti-IL-1 (anakinra) and anti-IL-6 receptor (tocilizumab) treatments have also been used to treat MAS successfully because these biologics help inhibit the action of the major proinflammatory cytokines produced during MAS.

6.4 INFLAMMATORY BOWEL DISEASE

IBD is an increasingly common chronic inflammatory condition. It encompasses specific conditions such as ulcerative colitis and Crohn's disease. The etiology of IBD is complex and is influenced by multiple genetic and environmental factors. For example, Crohn's disease currently has over 70 identified susceptibility genes, each of which confers a different level of risk in terms of developing the disease.

Within the North European and North American populations the occurrence of IBD is roughly 1 per 1000 of the population. However, the actual incidence varies quite dramatically between specific population groups consistent with the involvement of genetic factors in the initiation and the development of various forms of IBD. The development, propagation, and progression of IBD are also heavily influenced by interactions between the host and the intestinal microbiota—an interaction that is commonly disrupted and dysregulated in IBD. There are many causes and triggers for this dysregulation, which include infection, chronic inflammation, treatment (antibiotic)-induced perturbations of the commensal flora, dietary factors, environmental triggers, and genetic factors. Mutations in a number of the genes identified as susceptibility factors for IBD are connected with innate immune functions such as autophagy, PRR signaling, and the production and secretion of AMPs. Examples of affected genes include *NOD2*, *ATG16L1*, *CARD9*, *TCF4*, and *XBP1* among others.

At the functional level, many of the IBD-associated polymorphic changes in these genes alter Paneth cell function and therefore lead to alterations in either the production or the secretion of AMPs. This subsequently contributes to changes in the composition of the host microbiota, the efficiency with which pathogenic microbes can be combated, and ultimately tends to increase the inflammatory potential of the intestinal tract, thereby contributing to disease development and progression.

6.5 ANIMAL MODELS OF INFLAMMATORY DISORDERS

Interleukin-1α and interleukin-1β are often viewed as master regulators of inflammation. It is clear that human autoinflammatory diseases can result from the dysregulation of innate immune signaling pathways with myeloid cells often playing a crucial role in disease progression, presumably as a result of their functional role as first responders to danger. The importance of mutations in PRRs, such as NLRP3, NLRC4, and NOD2, is readily apparent and well studied. In addition, defects in other PRR pathways, for example, those that lead to STING activation following nucleic acid detection in the cytoplasm, can also induce autoinflammation and have been associated with increased cytokine secretion and enhanced disease severity for conditions including systemic lupus erythematosus, Aicardi–Goutieres syndrome, STING-associated vasculopathy with onset in infancy, and even the development of cancer.

The majority of these inflammatory conditions are pretty rare, which is obviously clinically desirable. It does, however, make understanding the molecular pathways leading to disease development and progression difficult to elucidate and study in a physiological context due to the limited availability of primary patient-derived cells to work with. Consequently, animal models provide an important pathway for working out the mechanisms of disease and the development of potential therapeutics. However, as we will see, there can also be a number of limitations with these models meaning that the data obtained require careful interpretation in relation to human pathogenesis.

As highlighted earlier the CAPS represent a spectrum of diseases that includes three major conditions. These are, in increasing order of severity: FCAS, MWS, and NOMID. Recently the groups of Hoffman and Strober generated the first murine models of the CAPS providing an opportunity for the detailed study and analysis of the mechanistic basis of these diseases in a whole organism. The development of disease in the animal model was broadly similar to that in humans but did not mimic all symptoms. The overall severity of the conditions was dramatically increased in mice and the order of disease severity was altered. In particular, mutations connected to FCAS were the most severe in mice and generally led to interuterine or perinatal lethality.

In humans, interleukin-1 inhibitors and antagonists have provided highly successful treatments for the CAPS consistent with the causative nature of enhanced IL-1β secretion resulting from NLRP3 hyperactivation. However, in the murine models the progression of disease was shown to only be partially dependent on IL-1β because introduction of the mutations for MWS and FCAS to mice lacking the IL-1R did not result in a loss of symptoms. Instead a Th17 response dominated the pathology. It is unclear if this Th17 phenotype is also responsible for the reversal in the order of disease severity, but it may well be a major contributing factor to the differences seen between the human and murine conditions.

Interleukin-18 secretion also results from activation and indeed autoactivation of NLRP3. Mice lacking the IL-18R but possessing FCAS-related NLRP3 mutations showed increased, but not statistically significant, survival rates. However, if instead these mice had an *Nlrp3* gene possessing an MWS-causing mutation, almost all mice survived to adulthood and showed limited clinical signs of disease. Together this suggests that IL-18 may have a particularly important role in the pathogenesis of MWS, particularly during the early stages of the disease.

The failure of mice to manifest an identical, or even anticipated, range of clinical symptoms in inflammatory disorders compared with human patients is not limited to the CAPS. Two recent pieces of work, one from the laboratory of Doug Golenbock and the other from the group of Michael Davey, have demonstrated that mice do not display comparable clinical symptoms, including inflammation, to humans when genetically engineered to develop pyogenic arthritis, pyoderma gangrenosum, and acne syndrome or Blau syndrome, respectively.

Nonsynonymous mutations in Proline-Serine-Threonine Phosphatase–interacting Protein-1 (PSTPIP1), such as A230T and E250Q, have been postulated to cause pyogenic arthritis, pyoderma gangrenosum, and acne syndrome. This may result from alterations in the interaction between PSTPIP1 and the inflammasome-forming protein Pyrin. This syndrome is characterized by joint destruction resulting from an early onset and recurrent sterile arthritis. In some cases patients can also develop cystic acne and skin ulceration. Successful treatment using the IL-1 antagonist anakinra is strongly supportive of the involvement of inflammatory pathways such as the inflammasome, as is the fact that monocytes from pyogenic arthritis, pyoderma gangrenosum, and acne syndrome patients secrete an enhanced level of IL-1β. However, while mice genetically deficient, or ectopically expressing the gain-of-function mutant A230T form of PSTPIP1, display increased levels of circulating cytokines, they failed to develop the most common symptoms of pyogenic arthritis, pyoderma gangrenosum, and acne syndrome, namely pyogenic arthritis and skin inflammation. Furthermore, mice ectopically expressing A230T PSTPIP1 showed no physical evidence supporting the development of arthritis and their joints lacked any synovial infiltration containing mono- or polymorphonuclear cells.

IL-1–driven inflammation is clearly important for the development and progression of pyogenic arthritis, pyoderma gangrenosum, and acne syndrome. However, PSTPIP1 deletion or mutation failed to disrupt either caspase-1–dependent inflammasome–mediated IL-1β secretion or sterile inflammation brought about by subcutaneous turpentine injection. This suggests that the role of PSTPIP1 gain-of-function mutants in the development of pyogenic arthritis, pyoderma gangrenosum, and acne syndrome is more complex than a simple disruption of inflammatory regulation. While this view is supported by the recent observation that not all individuals carrying PSTPIP1 gain-of-function mutants go on to develop pyogenic arthritis, pyoderma gangrenosum, and acne syndrome, the data from the murine model must also be viewed in light of the species differences in the relevant proteins. Specifically, murine Pyrin protein lacks the B30.2/Spry domain found within the human protein. As the region of Pyrin involved in interaction with PSTPIP1 is currently unknown, it remains plausible that under physiological conditions in the mouse that these two proteins do not interact and hence Pyrin functionality is unaffected by mutation of PSTPIP1. In humans the presence of the B30.2/Spry domain may dramatically alter the dynamics of protein interaction and consequently the impact of PSTPIP1 mutation on disease progression.

Blau syndrome is a rare autosomal dominant condition that results in uveitis, arthritis, and dermatitis due to granulomatous inflammation. It is caused by mutations in the central nucleotide-binding domain of NOD2. These mutations result in ligand-independent receptor hyperactivation leading to an increased basal activity of NFκB-mediated proinflammatory signaling pathways. These mutations have been mapped to two distinct regions of the NOD2 nucleotide-binding domain, namely helical domain 1 and the nucleotide and magnesium ion-binding pocket. This has resulted in the hypothesis that hyperactivation of NOD2 results from either disruption of the maintenance of an autoinhibited form of the receptor or is due to interference in the process of nucleotide binding and hydrolysis.

The rarity of Blau syndrome has meant that much of our understanding of how the disease manifests has resulted from the study of cell-based systems containing overexpressed Blau syndrome–associated NOD2 mutants. In these systems, disease-causing mutants are hyperactive in the absence of ligand stimulation but do not respond excessively to the presence of the NOD2 ligand muramyl dipeptide. To understand the mechanistic basis of Blau syndrome, Davey and coworkers have recently created a knock-in mouse containing an R314Q mutation in NOD2, analogous to the most common mutation observed in humans, R334Q. The knock-in nature of this mutant means that the NOD2 gene remains under the control of its endogenous promoter, and consequently the R314Q mutant NOD2 protein is expressed at levels comparable with those seen for wild-type receptor.

The R314Q NOD2 knock-in mice showed no evidence of increased cytokine production following either systemic or intraocular stimulation with muramyl dipeptide. Their wild-type counterparts respond robustly under these conditions. This pattern was also seen following the maturation and stimulation of murine bone marrow–derived macrophages and monocyte-derived macrophages obtained from Blau syndrome patients. In addition the homozygous Arg314Asn mutant NOD2 bone marrow–derived macrophages displayed no evidence of the degradation of inhibitors of NFκB signaling, or of the phosphorylation of members of the stress kinases. Arg314Asn NOD2 showed no alteration in transcriptional behavior but appeared to result in the truncation of NOD2 to a smaller 80 kDa form in the cell. How this occurs or what the implications on NOD2 function are, have yet to be determined. While the experimental evidence for a loss of NOD2 function in this model appears quite strong and clearly contrasts with the gain-of-function mechanistic phenotypes previously described, there remains one major caveat—the homozygous R314Q mutant NOD2 mouse failed to develop any symptoms consistent with the development of Blau syndrome. Clearly, more remains to be done to consolidate the in vivo, in vitro, and overexpression models of this autoinflammatory disorder. Certainly, given the locational proximity of the Blau syndrome and CAPS polymorphisms on the structures of NOD2 and NLRP3, respectively, it would be mechanistically intriguing should they have completely contrasting functional impacts.

The phenotypic differences between the murine models and the human patients, are not severe enough to bring into doubt the validity of their use as an experimental tool for studying the mechanisms of autoinflammatory disease. However, it does cause us to pause for thought and consider how exactly these, and other animal models, translate to the human patient. In particular, broader questions about the presence, or indeed absence, of additional cofactors involved in the signaling cascades need addressing as does the possibility that many of these diseases may in fact have a much more complex etiology than that, which results from a single genetic mutation.

REFERENCES AND FURTHER READING

Brydges SD, Broderick L, Mcgeough MD, Pena CA. Divergence of IL-1, IL-18, and cell death in NLRP3 inflammasomopathies. J Clin Invest 2013;123(11):4695–705.

Chinetti-Gbaguidi G, Colin S, Staels B. Macrophage subsets in atherosclerosis. Nat Rev Cardiol November 4, 2014;12(1):10–7.

Choy E. Understanding the dynamics: pathways involved in the pathogenesis of rheumatoid arthritis. Rheumatology July 1, 2012;51(Suppl. 5):v3–11.

Colin S, Chinetti-Gbaguidi G, Staels B. Macrophage phenotypes in atherosclerosis. Immunol Rev November 2014;262(1):153–66.

Danot O, Marquenet E, Vidal-Ingigliardi D, Richet E. Wheel of life, wheel of death: a mechanistic insight into signaling by STAND proteins. Structure February 13, 2009;17(2):172–82.

Dinarello CA, van der Meer JWM. Treating inflammation by blocking interleukin-1 in humans. Semin Immunol December 15, 2013;25(6):469–84. Elsevier Ltd.

Duewell P, Kono H, Rayner KJ, Sirois CM, Vladimer G, Bauernfeind FG, et al. NLRP3 inflammasomes are required for atherogenesis and activated by cholesterol crystals. Nature April 29, 2010;464(7293):1357–61.

Dugan J, Griffiths E, Snow P, Rosenzweig H, Lee E, Brown B, et al. Blau syndrome-associated Nod2 mutation alters expression of full-length NOD2 and limits responses to muramyl dipeptide in knock-in mice. J Immunol November 26, 2014.

Goh FG, Midwood KS. Intrinsic danger: activation of toll-like receptors in rheumatoid arthritis. Rheumatology January 1, 2012;51(1):7–23.

Grebe A, Latz E. Cholesterol crystals and inflammation. Curr Rheumatol Rep March 15, 2013;15(3):313.

Hu Z, Yan C, Liu P, Huang Z, Ma R, Zhang C, et al. Crystal structure of NLRC4 reveals its autoinhibition mechanism. Science July 12, 2013;341(6142):172–5.

Maekawa S, Ohto U, Shibata T, Miyake K, Shimizu T. Crystal structure of NOD2 and its implications in human disease. Nat Commun June 10, 2016;7:11813.

McInnes IB, Buckley CD, Isaacs JD. Cytokines in rheumatoid arthritis—shaping the immunological landscape. Nat Rev Rheumatol December 10, 2015;12(1):63–8.

Meng G, Zhang F, Fuss I, Kitani A, Strober W. A mutation in the Nlrp3 gene causing inflammasome hyperactivation potentiates Th17 cell-dominant immune responses. Immunity June 19, 2009;30(6):860–74. Elsevier Ltd.

Miceli-Richard C, Lesage S, Rybojad M, Prieur AM, Manouvrier-Hanu S, Häfner R, et al. CARD15 mutations in Blau syndrome. Nat Genet September 2001;29(1):19–20.

Mullen LM, Chamberlain G, Sacre S. Pattern recognition receptors as potential therapeutic targets in inflammatory rheumatic disease. Arthritis Res Ther December 15, 2015;17(1):122.

Parkhouse R, Boyle JP, Monie TP. Blau syndrome polymorphisms in NOD2 identify nucleotide hydrolysis and helical domain 1 as signalling regulators. FEBS Lett September 17, 2014;588(18):3382–9. Federation of European Biochemical Societies.

Peled M, Fisher EA. Dynamic aspects of macrophage polarization during atherosclerosis progression and regression. Front Immunol November 12, 2014;5.

Rajamäki K, Lappalainen J, Oörni K, Välimäki E, Matikainen S, Kovanen PT, et al. Cholesterol crystals activate the NLRP3 inflammasome in human macrophages: a novel link between cholesterol metabolism and inflammation. PLoS One 2010;5(7):e11765.

Schett G, Dayer J-M, Manger B. Interleukin-1 function and role in rheumatic disease. Nat Rev Rheumatol December 10, 2015;12(1):14–24.

Smolen JS, Aletaha D, McInnes IB. Rheumatoid arthritis. Lancet May 2016.

Sterba G, Sterba Y. Controlling inflammation. Dermatol Clin July 2013;31(3):507–11.

Thwaites R, Chamberlain G, Sacre S. Emerging role of endosomal toll-like receptors in rheumatoid arthritis. Front Immunol 2014;5.

Wang D, Höing S, Patterson HC, Ahmad UM, Rathinam VAK, Rajewsky K, et al. Inflammation in mice ectopically expressing human pyogenic arthritis, pyoderma gangrenosum, and acne (PAPA) syndrome-associated PSTPIP1 A230T mutant proteins. J Biol Chem February 15, 2013;288(7):4594–601.

Wright HL, Moots RJ, Bucknall RC, Edwards SW. Neutrophil function in inflammation and inflammatory diseases. Rheumatology September 1, 2010;49(9):1618–31.

Index

'*Note*: Page numbers followed by "f" indicate figures.'

A

Adaptive immune response
  APCs, 13
  complement
    B cells, function of, 175–177
    T-cell response, 177
  dendritic cell
    conventional and plasmacytoid, 180
    phagocytosis, 179–180
    T cells, 181–183
    types, 179–180
Aicardi–Goutières syndrome, 196–197
Antigen-presenting cells (APCs), 4–5
  lymph nodes, 16–17
  macrophages and dendritic cells, 19
Antimicrobial peptides (AMPs)
  cationic nature, 29
  defensins, 31
  indocilidin, 30–31
  peptide chains, 29
  structures of, 29, 30f
Apoptosis
  extrinsic apoptotic pathway, 112
  intrinsic apoptotic pathway, 110
  molecular process of, 110
  regulation and control of, 112–113
Atherosclerosis, 189–192
Autoinflammatory syndromes
  CAPSs, 198–199
  classical descriptions of, 196–197
  FMF, 197–198
  IL-1 family member antagonists, 199–201
  IL-1β, 197
  MAS, 199
  periodic inflammatory disorders, treatment of, 201–202
Autophagy
  innate immune responses, homeostatic functions involved in, 36–37
  T and B cells, 178–179

B

B cells
  autophagy, 178–179
  complement, 175–177
  lymphocytes, 20
Basophils, 54–55
Blood coagulation pathways, 98
Blood–brain barrier (BBB), 94

C

C4 binding protein (C4BP), 106
Caspase recruitment domains (CARDs), 108, 130
Caspases
  active sites of, 108
  caspase-12, 109
  caspase-8, 107–108
  pro-caspases, 108
  zymogens, 108
Cell death, 25–26
  apoptosis
    extrinsic apoptotic pathway, 112
    intrinsic apoptotic pathway, 110
    molecular process of, 110
    regulation and control of, 112–113
  necroptosis, 114
  necrosis, 113–114
  pyroptosis, 116
Commensal flora, 34–35
Complement system
  complement cascade, activation of
    alternative pathway, 100–102
    classical pathway, 102
    lectin pathway, 102–103
  C5 convertase, role of, 104
  disease, 106–107
  Gram-negative bacteria, 104–105
  inflammation and phagocyte recruitment, promotion of, 103–104
  MAC, formation of, 104
  regulation, 105–106
  target phagocytosis, stimulation of, 105

Complete Freunds' adjuvant (CFA),
185
C-reactive protein, 96
Cryopyrin-associated periodic syndromes
(CAPSs), 198–199
C-type lectin receptor (CLR) signaling
dectin-1, 71
dectin-2 and mincle, 71–72
inhibitory receptors, 72–73
ITAM, 70–71
structural domains, 70f
tyrosine-based activation motif–independent
signaling, 72
Cytokines
acute phase response and acute phase
proteins, 94–97
cell death
apoptosis, 110–113
necroptosis, 114
necrosis, 113–114
pyroptosis, 116
enzymatic cascades and enzymatic
activation
blood coagulation pathways, 98
caspases, 107–109
complement cascade, activation of,
100–107
eicosanoids, 99–100
GM-CSF, 93–94
IL-10, 92
IL-17 family, 92–93
IL-21, 92–93
IL-22, 92–93
IL-4 and IL-13, 92
IL-5, 92
IL-6, 89–90
IL-8, 90–91
interferon family, 87–89
interleukin-1 family
IL-18, 85
IL-1α and IL-1β, 85
IL-33 and -36, 85–86
proinflammatory nature of, 86–87
MCP1, 94
MIP, 94
ROS, 97–98
TGFβ, 94
TNF, 87
Cytoplasm, nucleic acid–sensing immune
receptors in
PYHIN receptor family, 78
RIG-I family, 77–78
STING and innate detection of,
78–79

D
Danger/damage-associated molecular patterns
(DAMPs), 95
Death domain (DD), 65
Deficiency in IL-1 receptor antagonist (DIRA),
199–201
Dendritic cell
conventional and plasmacytoid, 180
phagocytosis, 179–180
T cells, 181–183
types, 179–180

E
Eicosanoids, 99–100
Endoplasmic reticulum (ER), 36
Endosomal membrane, 127–129
Eosinophils
allergic and antihelminth immune processes,
53–54
cationic peptides and proteins, 52
cytokines and chemokines, 52
growth factors, 52–53
lipid mediators, 52
Erythrocytes, 17–18
nonmammalian vertebrates, 18
primary function of, 18

F
Familial mediterranean fever (FMF),
197–198
physiological cause of, 198–199
treatment of, 201–202
Flagellin
extracellular, TLR5, 149–152
intracellular
NAIP/NLRC4 inflammasome, 153,
154f, 155
LRRs, 153–155
ASC, 155
major immune stimulus, 149

G
Gamma-delta (γδ) T cells, 58–59
Gasdermin D, 116, 130
Granulocyte-macrophage colony-stimulating
factor (GM-CSF), 93–94
Gut-associated lymphoid tissue (GALT), 28

H
Hemagglutinin (HA), 156
H-ficolin, 102–103
Human leukocyte antigen (HLA), 171–172

I

Immune cells
  APCs, 19–20
  cell death, 25–26
  erythrocytes, 17–18
  granulocyte, 19
  leukocytes, 17–18
  lymphocytes and NK cells, 20–22
  monocytes, 19
  protein and peptide defenses, 22–25
Immunoglobulin A (IgA), 31–34
Immunoreceptor tyrosine-based activation
      motif (ITAM), 70–71
Inflammasome-based signaling, 76–77
Inflammatory bowel disease (IBD), 202–203
Inflammatory disorders, animal models of
  Arg314Asn mutant NOD2 mouse, 205–206
  Blau syndrome, 205
  CAPS, 203
  IL-1–driven inflammation, 204–205
  IL-1α and IL-1β, 203
  interleukin-18, 204
  PSTPIP1, 204
Influenza A virus (IAV)
  antigenic drift and antigenic shift, 159
  antiviral signaling pathways, activation of, 162
  direct antiviral activity, 162
  evasion of, 164
  NLRs, 162–163
  noncanonical inflammasome formation, 162
  replication cycle of, 156–159
  RIG-I, molecular basis of, 160
  RLRs, 160
  TLRs, 160
Innate immune response
  dendritic cell, 179–183
    conventional and plasmacytoid, 180
    phagocytosis, 179–180
    T cells, 181–183
    types, 179–180
  IAV
    antigenic drift and antigenic shift, 159
    antiviral signaling pathways, activation
        of, 162
    direct antiviral activity, 162
    evasion of, 164
    NLRs, 162–163
    noncanonical inflammasome formation, 162
    replication cycle of, 156–159
    RIG-I, molecular basis of, 160
    RLRs, 160
    TLRs, 160
  Salmonella, bacterial infection. *See*
      Salmonella, bacterial infection

Innate immune system
  autoinflammatory syndromes
    CAPSs, 198–199
    classical descriptions of, 196–197
    FMF, 197–198
    IL-1 family member antagonists,
        199–201
    IL-1β, 197
    MAS, 199
    periodic inflammatory disorders,
        treatment of, 201–202
  brief history of
    adaptive response, 1
    danger theory, 8–10, 9f
    immunological timeline, 2f
    infectious nonself, detection of, 5f
    innate response, 1
    NFκB, 6
    PAMP, 4–5
    phagocytic cells, 2–4
    PRRs, 4–7
    self–nonself theory, 7–8
    T and B cells, 4
    TLR4, 6
  cellular basis of
    dendritic cells, 46–47
    eosinophils, 52–54
    gamma-delta (γδ) T cells, 58–59
    innate lymphoid cells, 55–58
    macrophages, 42–46
    mast cells and basophils, 54–55
    monocytes, 42
    neutrophils, 47–51
  complex defense system
    adaptive response, 10–12, 12f
    innate response, 10–12, 12f
    T and B cells, 13
  functional elements
    barrier functions, 15–16
    categories, 13
    fever therapy, 15
    immune cells, 17–22
    immune tissues, 16–17
    inflammation, cardinal elements of,
        14–15
  homeostatic functions
    autophagy, 36–37
    heat shock response, 36
    UPR, 36
  IBD, 202–203
  inflammation and atherosclerosis
    cholesterol crystals, 192
    macrophages and pathogenesis, 190, 192
    oxLDL, 190

Innate immune system (*continued*)
  inflammatory disorders, animal models of
    Arg314Asn mutant NOD2 mouse,
      205–206
    Blau syndrome, 205
    CAPS, 203
    IL-1–driven inflammation, 204–205
    IL-1α and IL-1β, 203
    interleukin-18, 204
    PSTPIP1, 204
  mucosa-associated
    gastrointestinal tract, 26–28
    Peyer's patches and M cells, 28
    secreted defenses, 28–35
  pattern recognition receptor signaling
    pathways
    CLR signaling, 70–73
    cytoplasm, nucleic acid–sensing immune
      receptors in, 77–79
    cytoplasmic detection, 73
    domain organization of, 61–62
    exogenous and endogenous dangers,
      59–61
    NLRs, 73–77
    TLRs, 62–69
  RA
    etiology of, 194
    initiation and establishment of, 194
    pathogenesis of, 195
    proinflammatory cytokines,
      195–196
    PRRs, 195–196
Innate lymphoid cells (ILCs), 21
  NK cells, 55–57
  type I, 57
  type II, 58
  type III, 58
Integrated innate immunity
  bacterial lipopolysaccharide, detection of
    BB loop, 126–127
    extracellular, 123–126
    Gram-negative bacterial infection, 121
    intracellular LPS, 130
    KDO, 123
    lipid A, 123
    MD-2:TLR4:LPS complexes, 126–127
    plasma membrane and endosomal
      membrane, 127–129
  innate response
    IAV, 155–164
    Salmonella, bacterial infection. *See*
      Salmonella, bacterial infection
  interleukin 1β, inflammasome

    inflammasome activation, 132–140
    protein interactions, 140
    regulation of, 141–144
Interferon-stimulated genes (ISGs), 89
Interleukin 1β, inflammasome
  inflammasome activation
    AIM2, 135–137
    NAIP/NLRC4, 135
    NLRP1, 135
    NLRP3, 137–140
    proinflammatory complex, 133
  protein interactions, 140
  regulation of, 141–144

L

Laboratory of genetics and physiology 2
  (LGP2), 77
Leucine-rich repeats (LRRs), 133–135
L-ficolin, 102–103
Licensed adjuvants, 183–184
  alum, 184
  muramyl dipeptide, 185
  nucleic acids, 185
  oil-and-water emulsions, 184
Lipopolysaccharide (LPS), 6
  BB loop, 126–127
  extracellular
    molecular interactions, 126
    structural basis of, 125f
    TLR4 signaling, activation of,
      123–126
  Gram-negative bacterial infection, 121
  intracellular LPS, 130
  KDO, 123
  lipid A, 123
  MD-2:TLR4:LPS complexes, 126–127
  plasma membrane and endosomal
    membrane, 127–129
Lymph nodes, 16
  APCs, 16–17
Lymphoid organs
  primary, 16
  secondary, 16
    MALT, 17
    spleen, 17
    tonsils, 17

M

Macrophage activation syndrome (MAS), 199
Macrophage inflammatory protein (MIP), 94
Macrophages
  monocyte-derived macrophages, 43

neutrophil extravasation
  adhesion, 49–50
  crawling, 50–51
  neutrophil-driven bacterial killing, 51
  rolling, 49
  transmigration, 51
tissue-resident macrophages, 43–44
Major histocompatibility complex (MHC)
    class I, 56–57
  class I genes, transcriptional regulation
    expression of, 171–172
    NLRC5, 172
  class II genes, transcriptional regulation
    CIITA, 174–175
    expression of, 171–172
Mannose-binding lectin (MBL), 102–103
Mast cells, 54–55
Melanoma differentiation associated 5
    (MDA5), 77
Mixed-lineage kinase domain-like protein
    (MLKL), 114
Monocytes, 42
Mucosa-associated lymphoid tissue (MALT), 16
Muramyl dipeptide (MDP), 74, 135, 185
Myddosome complex
  DD, 65
  formation of, 65–69
  IRAK family, 65–69

N

Natural killer (NK) cells, 20–22, 172
Necroptosis, 114
Necroptotic cell death pathway, 115f
Necrosis, 113–114
Neutrophil extracellular traps (NETs), 51
Nuclear factor kappa B (NFκB), 6
Nucleotide-binding, leucine-rich repeat–
    containing receptors (NLRs)
  inflammasome-based signaling, 76–77
  NOD1 and NOD2 receptor signaling,
    74–76

P

Pathogen-associated molecular patterns
    (PAMPs), 4–5, 51, 95
Pattern recognition receptors (PRRs) signaling
    pathways
  alum, 184
  CLR signaling
    dectin-1, 71
    dectin-2 and mincle, 71–72
    inhibitory receptors, 72–73

ITAM, 70–71
    structural domains, 70f
    tyrosine-based activation motif–
      independent signaling, 72
  cytoplasm, nucleic acid–sensing immune
      receptors in, 77–79
  cytoplasmic detection, 73
  DAMPs and PAMPs, 95
  domain organization of, 61–62
  exogenous and endogenous dangers, 59–61
  IL-8, 91
  muramyl dipeptide, 185
  NLRs, 73–77
  nucleic acids, 185
  oil-and-water emulsions, 184
  Salmonella, 145
  TLRs
    myddosome complex, 65–69
    plasma and endosomal membrane, 62–64
Plasma membrane, 127–129
Protein and peptide defenses
  complement system
    basic level, 23–24
    enzymatic cascade pathways, 24
  cytokines, 25
  pattern recognition, 22–23
Protein C thrombomodulin system, 98
Pyroptotic cell death, 116

R

Reactive oxygen species (ROS), 51, 97–98
Rheumatoid arthritis (RA)
  etiology of, 194
  initiation and establishment of, 194
  pathogenesis of, 195
  proinflammatory cytokines, 195–196
  PRRs, 195–196

S

Salmonella bongori, 144
Salmonella enterica, 144
Salmonella, bacterial infection
  flagellin
    extracellular, TLR5, 149–152
    intracellular, 153–155
    major immune stimulus, 149
  innate immune components
    PRRs, 145–146
    trigger method, 145
  lipoproteins stimulate TLR2-driven
    inflammatory signaling, 146–149
Salmonellosis, 144–145

Scavenger receptor A (SR-A), 190
Serum amyloid A, 97
Systemic lupus erythematosus (SLE), 107

T

T-cell receptor (TCR), 58
  autophagy, 178–179
  complement, 177
  dendritic cells interact, 181–183
  lymphocytes, 20
Toll/interleukin-1 resistance (TIR), 126–127
Toll-like receptor (TLR) signaling pathways
  BB loop, 126–127
  extracellular LPS, 123–126

MD-2:TLR4:LPS complexes, 126–127
myddosome complex, 65–69
plasma and endosomal membrane, 62–64
plasma membrane and endosomal
    membrane, 127–129
Transforming growth factor beta (TGFβ), 94
Tumor necrosis factor (TNF), 87

U

Unfolded protein response (UPR), 36

V

Vaccination, 183–185